María de Lourdes Alonso Spilsbury

Animal welfare

María de Lourdes Alonso Spilsbury

Animal welfare

An ethical approach to meat consumption from the perspective of veterinary medicine and zootechnics.

Imprint

Any brand names and product names mentioned in this book are subject to trademark, brand or patent protection and are trademarks or registered trademarks of their respective holders. The use of brand names, product names, common names, trade names, product descriptions etc. even without a particular marking in this work is in no way to be construed to mean that such names may be regarded as unrestricted in respect of trademark and brand protection legislation and could thus be used by anyone.

Cover image: www.ingimage.com

This book is a translation from the original published under ISBN 978-620-0-34879-1.

Publisher:
Sciencia Scripts
is a trademark of
Dodo Books Indian Ocean Ltd. and OmniScriptum S.R.L publishing group

120 High Road, East Finchley, London, N2 9ED, United Kingdom
Str. Armeneasca 28/1, office 1, Chisinau MD-2012, Republic of Moldova, Europe
Printed at: see last page
ISBN: 978-620-6-85552-1

Without animal protein, it is very likely that we would not be as we are - since the last 200,000 years - as the archaeological remains of the hominids that preceded us indicate. Increasingly, however, animal rights activist movements as well as individual vegetarians are advocating for a supposedly green planet in which no meat and, in some cases, no animal products are consumed. However, according to the FAO (2013), around 1.3 billion people in the world live from livestock farming, of which 987 million are poor.

In the practice of teaching ethics and animal welfare to students of veterinary medicine and zootechnics (MVZ) in the second trimester of the degree, I have noticed that several of them take positions against the handling of animals due to a personal bias because they are animal rights activists, but lack the arguments either for or against their use, let alone their use for the production of animal protein for human consumption.

This essay finds its justification in the need to provide ethical and scientific arguments to meat consumers, defending their food autonomy in the face of the moral conflict that this behaviour causes in society, being criticised and sometimes attacked by activists, ovo-lacto-vegetarians or vegetarians, whose eating habits show ethical and moral respect for animals, by refusing to eat meat and animal products, but a lack of respect for those who do consume them.

Another objective of this manuscript is to provide a framework on the use of contemporary ethical principles and theories on our relationship with food animals - such as teleological theories, deontological theories and principlism, among others - that the MVZ student can understand as an acquisition of instrumental competences, and apply it to the dilemma of meat consumption.

Supported by documentary information with abundant bibliography, this paper analyses the meat-eating dilemma, with arguments from philosophy, ethics, anthropology, animal welfare science, applied ethology, nutrition, psychology and sustainability. A shorter version of this essay was submitted for the Diploma in Bioethics by the College of Bioethics in Mexico City in November 2013.

For ease of reading, the manuscript is divided into three sections. The first part examines the scientific arguments against the two main ethical objections to meat consumption: (a) the unnecessary killing of sentient beings, from the viewpoint of ***consequentialist or teleological theories*** ^ *and* animal rights, and

(b) the opposition to certain zootechnical practices surrounding meat production, which I address from the techno-scientific point of view - as a specialist in the area of pig production and applied ethology - by appealing to the deontological theories of our profession and the science of animal welfare.

In a second section, in addition to analysing the principles and theories that ethically or morally condemn the consumption of meat, under the assumption that meat is not necessary in the human diet, the phylogenic, ontogenetic, proximate (control and motivational mechanisms) and ultimate (adaptive function or advantage) causes of meat-eating behaviour are reasoned under the criteria of the ethologist Nikolas Tinbergen.

Aware that intensive animal production is involved with negative effects on the health of the ecosystem, animals and humans, the third and final part briefly discusses the issue of environmental ethics and sustainability, offering some alternatives to the meat consumption that mainly governs Western society.

Mexico City, June 2019.

---

[1] Consequentialist or teleological theories: from the Greek *telos,* meaning consequence, end or purpose. Ethical theories that emphasise goodness and badness, i.e. the results of actions (Rollin, BE. 2006, *Introduction to Veterinary Medical Ethics. Theory and Cases.* Zaragoza: Acribia, p. 23). The most famous of the consequentialist ethics is utilitarian ethics.

INTRODUCTION

Why did eating meat suddenly become an "ethical-ecological crime"? According to critics, including vegetarians, animal rights activists, as well as scientists who follow the animal liberation movement *(e.g.* Goodall and Bekoff, 2009), and particularly some contemporary philosophers (*e.g.* Regan, 1999; Rowlands, 1999; Singer, 1999), *"eating meat is immoral".* Yet, in general, people enjoy eating meat and most consider using animals for food production or science to be vitally necessary for our species (Harnad, 2018). In this essay, however, I will attempt to answer the objections to meat consumption.

First of all, I would like to start the controversy with the definition of the object of controversy to defend my position, *meat* is the skeletal muscle tissue, which represents about 35% to 65% of the carcass weight[2] of animals (mammals and birds) together with variable amounts of tissues that are attached to these muscles: connective tissue (ligaments, cartilage), nervous, adipose, bone and cartilage (Prandl, 1994); it is at the same time, the edible portion of healthy animals intended for human consumption (Ponce, 2010b). It also includes some animal organs (brain, tongue, heart, diaphragm, liver, etc.). With regard to its regulatory connotation in Mexico, *"meat is the structure composed of striated muscle fibre, whether or not accompanied by elastic connective tissue, fat, nerve fibres, lymphatic and blood vessels of animal species authorised for human consumption"* (NOM-009-Z00-1994). When referring to meat consumption in this essay, the emphasis will be on meat from domestic animals considered as food animals[3] .

While among the detractors of meat consumption, writers such as Robert Louis Stevenson (Stevenson, 2013), and Nobel Prize winners John Maxwell Coetzee (Coetzee, 2003) and Sir George Bernard Shaw[4] , allude in their respective works

---

[2] Carcass: Slaughtered animal, eviscerated, without head and without the distal part of the locomotive limbs (Oteyza, J. and Carmona, JR. 1985. *Diccionario de Zootecnia.* Mexico: Trillas, p. 49).

[3] Animals for slaughter: NOM-009-200-1994 defines them as *"those destined for slaughter, such as cattle, goats, pigs, poultry, horses or any other species destined for human consumption".*

[4] George Bernard Shaw, playwright (1856-1950). His position, succinctly stated, after he became a strict vegetarian at the age of 25 (in 1881), was *"A man of my spiritual intensity does not eat corpses".* An extract from his diaries reads: *"My situation is a solemn one. Life is offered to me on condition of eating beefsteaks. But death is better than cannibalism. My will contains directions for my funeral, which will be followed not by mourning coaches, but by oxen, sheep, flocks of poultry, and a small travelling aquarium of live fish, all wearing white scarves in honour of the man who perished rather than eat his fellow creatures". "A mind of the calibre of mine cannot derive its nutriment from cows".*

to the fact that man feeds on corpses. In this regard, I would like to comment on the following by appealing to the *fallacy of the "straw man"*[5] , as I think it is incorrect to exaggerate the exaggeration with which some philosophers and doctors *(e.g.* Singer, 1998, Vinyes, 2005; Plutarch, 2008) want to shame us meat eaters by resorting to such a judgement. I start from the premise that, from a scientific point of view, human beings are omnivores, we are not carnivores and much less scavengers; a corpse is a dead body without burial and with maggots. [It should be clarified that Plutarch, unlike the other characters cited, was not a vegetarian].

Available at: ivu.org/history/shaw/diaries.html

[5] Straw man fallacy: This consists of caricaturing the opponent's arguments or position, twisting their words or changing their meaning to facilitate a linguistic or dialectical attack. Its name alludes to the fact that the arguer does not combat the opposing arguments, but rather a false and vulnerable imitation of them, in order to give the illusion of defeating them easily (Wikipedia, 2013).

1. Moral implications of intensive food animal production and animal welfare as an ethical alternative

1.1 Moral consideration of animals

Deserving moral consideration would make the difference between being considered as an end in itself or, on the contrary, being treated in a purely instrumental way; in this respect, there are more than a thousand published works on the moral consideration of animals (Dorado, 2010). Current *zoocentric theories*[6] hold that all animals are worthy of moral consideration, from the most developed mammal to the simplest bacterium *(biocentric theory*[7] *)*, and are in line with Paul W. Taylor (2005), a proponent of biocentric ethics, who proposes that animals have *inherent worth*[8] '.

The contemporary philosopher Peter Singer (1999), on the other hand, does not consider that animals have rights and proposes their liberation; although he does refer to the acquisition of certain interests, and presents an *extended utilitarian ethic*[9] that seeks to satisfy the interests of the greatest possible number of vertebrates. Singer thinks that it is wrong to consider human life as more

---

[6] Zoocentric theories: These include the human being and the rest of the non-human animal species as a central reference (Sánchez, MA. 2002. The current ethical debate on the relationship between humans and animals. In: Lacadena, JR (ed.), *Los Derechos de los Animales.* Madrid: Universidad Pontificia Comillas, p. 110.)

[7] Biocentric theory: It focuses its moral consideration on all living beings. From the perspective of an egalitarian biocentric theory, coined by Paul W. Taylor (1981. The ethics for respect for nature. *Environon. Ethics,* 3 (3): 197-218), "we have *prima facie* moral obligations to plants and wild animals, members of the earth's biotic community. We are morally obligated *(ceteris paribus)* to protect or promote their good for *their own sake"* [An English translation of this essay, by Jorge Issa, can be found in Taylor, PW. 1998. The ethics of respect for nature. In: Kwiatkowska, T. and Issa, J. (eds.), *Los Caminos de la Ética Ambiental. An Anthology of Contemporary Texts.* Mexico: CONACyT, UAM, Plaza y Valdés, pp. 269-287]. Taylor's position is somewhat radical, as he considers that nature can perfectly well do without the human species.

[8] Inherent worth' presupposes the 'principle of moral consideration' according to which '[...] *insofar as an individual is an entity that has its own good, it deserves consideration';* but also the 'principle of intrinsic value' according to which '[...] *if an entity belongs to the community of life on Earth, regardless of what kind of entity it is in other respects, the realisation of its good is intrinsically valuable'.* [Taken from Taylor, PW. 2005. *The Ethics of Respect for Nature.* Presentation by Margarita M. Valdés. Trans. by Miguel Ángel Fernández Vargas. Mexico: UNAM, Instituto de Investigaciones Filosóficas, Cuadernos de Crítica 52, p. 15]. Inherent worth is independent of the merits of individuals or organisms, it does not depend on the opinion of others.

[9] Utilitarian ethics: Classical utilitarianism, as expounded by the founding father of utilitarianism, Jeremy Bentham, and refined by later philosophers such as John Stuart Mill and Henry Sidwick, judges actions by their tendency to maximise pleasure or happiness and minimise pain or unhappiness. [Taken from Singer, 1998, Animals and the value of life. In: Kwiatkowska, T. and Issa, J. *op. cit.,* p. 222].

important than animal life; however, in his extended utilitarian vision, he tries to level all rights, human and non-human.

It is not my intention in this manuscript to discuss the moral or arbitrary considerations that different authors may point out (see review by Dorado, 2010), rather, I start from the premise that it is not necessary to include animals in the moral community to protect their interests, as this is an ethical duty of all those of us who dedicate ourselves to veterinary medicine and zootechnics (MVZ), as stipulated in the "professional oath" in our Code of Professional Ethics[10][11] in Mexico (FedMVZ, 1999). In this order of ideas, I would like to take up Jeremy Bentham (1836) who coined the term deontology in 1832, thus exposing a way of looking at ethics in terms of the duties and obligations that professionals of a given discipline have. Likewise, I rely on the position of **contractualism**[1] of the philosopher John Rawls (2011), who has the advantage of avoiding paradoxes derived from including animals in the moral community, and maintains the position of accepting only indirect duties towards non-human animals. It is worth mentioning that although non-human animals are not moral agents, they are considered **moral patients**[1] as they suffer the effects and pay the price for many of our actions (Mosterín, 2007).

I must emphasise that in our profession we do not at any time disavow that animals are sentient beings, and rather we have every reason to consider them so, based on proven scientific knowledge - at least in vertebrates - that they possess the anatomical structures and mechanisms necessary to generate emotions (Darwin, 1984; Boissy *et al.*, 2007; Balcombe, 2009) and feelings (*e.g.* Broom, 1998), as well as consciousness (Rollin, 1986, 1989; Dol, 1999). Personally, I would also appeal to **emotivism**"[3] as a moral theory of empathy towards animal care; to paraphrase the philosopher Jesús Mosterín, *"our intuitions and emotions and moral feelings are the touchstone of ethical theories, and not the other way around". "It is good feelings that move a growing number*

---

[10] The Code of Professional Ethics of the Veterinary Zootechnician in Mexico, 1999 version, of the Federation of Colleges and Associations of MVZ A. C., states in its Professional Oath: *'...I will strive to increase to the maximum extent possible the production of food of animal origin for the benefit of mankind, to safeguard human health by avoiding diseases that animals can transmit to them, and to avoid unnecessary suffering of these".*

[11] In animal ethics, the idea of contractualism is often used as a reason to exclude animals from the category of those with moral value in the individualistic sense (Croney, CC.; Gardner, B. & Baggot, S. 2004. Beyond animal husbandry: The study of farm animal cognition and ensuing ethical issues. *Essays in Philos.*, 5 (2): Article 8).

of good people to sympathise with animals and to mobilise in their defence" (Mosterín, 2007).

In this context, philosophy and bioethics expert Bernard E. Rollin has called upon veterinarians, scientific researchers, biologists, animal producers, and other groups involved in direct work with animals to review their professional actions and decisions, in order to give an eminently practical sense to a social ethics applied to the human-animal relationship in the daily context.

1.2 Animal interests and animal welfare

Rollin (1992) argues that we have reason to consider animals as ends in themselves, given that they show interests in, for example, food, sex and welfare, and that the difference between man and animal is, in this case, merely a difference of degree.

When talking about domestic animals, it must be taken into account that they should be able to thrive, have normal levels of growth and reproduction, and be reasonably free of disease, injury, malnutrition, and behavioural and physiological abnormalities. This is considered to be the biological functioning of the species, a criterion that is taken into account under the ***animal welfare*** approach[4] , a discipline that arose precisely as a scientific response to the demands made by lay people for the treatment of domestic animals in food production in the 1960s (Brambell Report, 1965). Moreover, the World Organisation for Animal Health (OIE, 2004) now recognises that animal welfare is a complex and multifaceted issue of general interest, with important scientific, ethical, economic and political dimensions.

Broom and Johnson (1993) indicate that animal welfare is a measurable state, it is a property of the animal and not something that is provided; it is not a characteristic that simply exists or not, but it presents a gradation ranging from very poor (bad) to very good, as for example, health. Therefore, to use the concept of animal welfare in a scientific way, it is always necessary to specify its level and not just its presence or absence; thus, an animal's level of welfare is poor when It has difficulty coping with changes in the environment or when it fails to do so, with pain and suffering being manifestations of limited welfare (Broom, 2004). And it is precisely the fact that animals may suffer that is sufficient reason to have a moral obligation not to harm them, which is known as the ***principle of***

non-maleficence[12] (Beauchamp and Childress, 1999; cited by Vanda, 2007).

The definition coined by the World Organisation for Animal Health integrates the three approaches to animal welfare, namely those related to functioning, affective or emotional state, and the ability to live a reasonably natural life and to be able to express natural behaviour. For this organisation, *"animal welfare refers to the way in which an animal copes with the conditions of its environment. An animal is in good welfare condition if it is healthy, comfortable, well fed, safe, able to express innate forms of behaviour, and free from unpleasant feelings of pain, fear or distress"* (OIE, 2008).

The scientific study of animal welfare has undergone unexpected developments over the last twenty-five years. There are now a number of scientists involved in quantifying animal welfare who accept that the level of welfare can get better or worse. For Broom (2004, 2010), *"it is therefore illogical to try to use the concept of welfare as an absolute state or to limit the term to the positive end of the scale; measurement and interpretation must be done objectively, and once welfare has been described, ethical decisions can be made"*.

The assessment of animal welfare status

The Five Freedoms (**Table 1**) derived from the Brambell Report (1965) have for several decades now been the source of reference for guidelines and/or codes of practice for various organisations around the world, including the OIE. Emphasis is also placed on the use of the Five Freedoms or Needs of Animals (FAWC, 1993) as indicators of animal welfare in the teaching of animal welfare in veterinary schools, which is undoubtedly the framework most widely used by scientists worldwide to assess animal welfare.

---

[12] Principle of non-maleficence: This is generally explained through the concept of harm. Beauchamp and Childress define it as follows: *"the word harm refers to that action of hindering, hindering or preventing the interests of one party from being fulfilled by causes including the self-injurious conditions and acts (intentional or unintentional) of the other party" (Beauchamp, TL and Childress, JF. 1999).* (Beauchamp, TL and Childress, JF. 1999. *Principles of Biomedical Ethics*. Spain: Masson. 4th ed., 522 pp.).

Box 1. The Five Animal Freedoms	
1	Freedom from hunger and thirst.
2	Freedom from discomfort.
3	Freedom from pain, injury or illness.
4	Freedom to express normal behaviour.
5	Freedom from fear and anxiety.
	Source: FAWC (1993).

The Five Freedoms can be approached from the **principled** proposal[13] of Beauchamp and Childress (1999), according to the criteria proposed by our colleague Beatriz Vanda (2013) -pathologist and specialist in bioethics- as follows: the principle of *non-harming* implies not causing them physical or mental suffering, that they are not hungry or thirsty and that they are kept with a minimum of stress and pain; the principle of *justice:* corresponds to feeding them according to their requirements, caring for their health, attending to them if they are sick or injured, and allowing them to express important natural behaviours; while that *of beneficence* would be to provide animals with environmental enrichment, advice and care by veterinarians as a moral responsibility. As can be seen in **Table 2**, principled ethics are implicit in the Five Freedoms of the FAWC (1993).

---

[13] Beauchamp and Childress (1999) present a list of moral principles which, in their view, have served to construct most of the codes of contemporary medical ethics, but a moment's reflection reveals that they actually go beyond this and are applicable to most human transactions, such as, for example, the behaviour of a teacher towards his or her students (Excerpt from Kraus, A. and Pérez Tamayo, R. 2007. *Diccionario Incompleto de Bioética con Comentarios y Preguntas.* Mexico: Taurus, pp. 170-171).

Table 2. Provisions to the Five Freedoms

Cinco Libertades	Provisiones
1: Sin sed, hambre, ni desnutrición	Acceso a agua fresca y dieta para mantener completa salud y vigor.
2: Sin confort y exposición al ambiente	Proveer ambiente apropiado incluyendo refugio y área confortable para descansar.
3: Sin dolor, daño, ni enfermedad	Mediante la prevención, diagnóstico y tratamiento oportunos.
4: Sin miedo, ni diestrés	Asegurar condiciones y tratamiento que eviten el sufrimiento mental.
5: Expresar el comportamiento normal	Mediante la provisión de espacio suficiente, instalaciones apropiadas y compañía de animales de su propia clase.

Source: FAWC (1993).

Animal welfare criteria have been refined over time, so that nowadays there are different assessment methods for farm animals [see reviews by Johnsen *et al.* (2001) and Alonso (2012ab)] that include indicators of health, behaviour and productive performance (Broom, 1991; Appleby *et al,* 2004; Mellor and Stafford, 2004; Perry, 2004; Weeks and Butterworth, 2004; Lagger, 2006; Smulders *et al.,* 2006; Broom and Fraser, 2007; Velarde and Geers, 2007; Vessier *et al.,* 2008; Mounier *et al,* 2010), as well as physiological indicators *(e.g.* Mormede *et al.,* 2007; Palme, 2012), and those related to the emotional states[14] of the animals *(e.g.* Wemelsfelder and Lawrence, 2001; Désire *et al.,* 2002; McMillan, 2005).

One way to assess emotional states is by recognising facial expressions in animals (Dalla Costa *et al.,* 2014; Gleerup *et al.,* 2014; Giminiani *et al.,* 2016; Leach and Descovich, 2016; Descovich et *al.,* 2017) or by the use of so-called

Qualitative Behavioural Assessment (QBA*).* For this purpose, measurement scales exist, for example for pigs (Reimert *et al.,* 2016), sheep (Richmond *et al.,* 2016), goats (Grosso *et al.,* 2014), calves (Brscic *et al.,* 2016) and horses (Dai *et*

---

[14] Dr. Marian S. Dawkins defines emotional states as those induced by positive or negative reinforcement, and may be accompanied by subjective feelings of pleasure or suffering, although not necessarily so (Dawkins, MS. 2008. The science of animal suffering. *Ethol.,* 114 (10): 937-945).

al., 2016), among other species.

To measure positive mental states supported by neurobiological studies, play is assessed as an indicator of good welfare (Held, 2016; Lidfors and Broekman, 2016; Rushen and de Passille, 2016). Other behavioural markers are the animals' vocalisations or acoustic signals (Baciadonna *et al.,* 2016; Briefer *et al.,* 2016; Friel *et al.,* 2016; Stomp *et al.,* 2018). In contrast, negative mental states are measured as an example by assessing the state of anhedonia[15] (Fureix, 2016).

Other non-invasive ways of assessing mental states include telemetry measurements, for example, heart rate variability (Baciadonna *et al.,* 2016; Marchant-Forde, 2016; Tamioso *et al.,* 2016; Byrd *etal.,* 2017), or skin or eye surface temperature, through the use of infra-red thermography (Rebelo *et al.,* 2014b; Herborn *et al.,* 2016; Telkanranta *et al.,* 2018).

Recently, Mellor (2016) proposed the "Five Domains Model", structured to assess particular physical and functional imbalances and constraints in the behavioural expression of animals, and identify the negative effects that the disruption, imbalance or constraint may have on them. The model incorporates four predominantly physical/functional domains: nutrition, environment, health and behaviour, and a mental domain, which focuses on all identified negative effects on the individual and their overall cumulative impact on welfare (Mellor and Beausoleil, 2015). The Five Domains Model goes beyond the provision of the Five Freedoms by minimising negative experiences while providing animals with opportunities for positive experiences, i.e. providing them with a *"life worth living"* (Mellor, 2016); thus, quality of life is the new paradigm in animal welfare.

The development of food security, sustainability and humane strategies requires the implementation of animal welfare guidelines, research and development in the practical improvement of on-farm management and welfare, as well as knowledge transfer to the farmer (Appleby, 2017). At the international level, the World Bank's International Finance Corporation (IFC) has recognised that animal welfare is an important element in animal production worldwide and that ensuring animal welfare increases the economic profitability of livestock farms (Galindo and Manteca, 2016). Moreover, audits have been shown to improve animal

---

[15] Anhedonia: in humans is defined as a marked decrease in interest or pleasure in any activity. It is a common symptom of mood disorders associated with negative affective states such as clinical depression and post-traumatic stress disorder.

welfare in the long run (Grandin, 2006).

To date, several on-farm and slaughterhouse animal welfare status assessment tools exist for almost all domestic species: pigs, dairy and beef cattle, and poultry and chickens; all of them from the Welfare Quality® project (2009abc) are available on the project's website (www.welfarequality.net). This European research project started in May 2004 and ended in 2009, funded by the European Commission with a budget of €14.4 million. It consists of a consortium of 44 partners (institutions and universities), representing 13 European countries and 4 in Latin America (Brazil, Chile, Mexico and Uruguay), with the participation of 450 scientists with expertise in the fields of biology, animal production and social sciences. The assessments recommended by this consortium are based on reliable and valid measurements, recorded by behavioural and animal health observations (Cozzi *et al.,* 2008), tested in more than 1,000 farms in nine EU countries and some Latin American countries.

Similarly, there are feasible, practical and valid protocols for assessing welfare in sheep, goats in extensive and intensive dairy systems, sport horses, working donkeys and turkeys under intensive farming systems - the predominant systems in the European Union - published by AWIN (*Animal Welfare Indicators*) (AWIN, 2015a-e). In this project - whose scientific coordinator is Dr. Adoaldo Zanella - four packages with practical *smartphone* applications have been developed to assess pain and recognise pain in farm conditions (Zanella *et al.,* 2015), with emphasis on assessing and mitigating pain in ewes and ewe lambs with mastitis, pregnancy toxaemia (Rebelo *et al.,* 2014a) and barking (Rebelo *et al.,* 2014b); measurements and pain control during castration of lambs, disbudding and disbudding of kids, as well as assessment of laminitis and post-castration pain in horses (Stucke *et al.,* 2014). The English version is available as pdf files and is also freely available (http://www.animal-welfare-indicators.net/site/). The AWIN project took two years and involved 142 scientists working in 11 institutions in nine countries and was sponsored by the European Commission at a cost of €6 million (Zanella *et al.,* 2015).

There are also OIE standards (2006) for the transport of animals for human consumption. This is undoubtedly the phase where the animals suffer the most welfare problems, as the Five Freedoms are affected: 1) no fresh water or food during the journey, even for 24 hours; 2) they suffer injuries during loading, journey and unloading; 3) they do not have enough space or the possibility of comfortable rest; 4) they suffer inadequate treatment; transport is an unknown event; and 5) they are overcrowded with few opportunities to express behaviours (Gallo, 2015).

1.3 Sentient beings

It is now widely accepted that vertebrate animals are sentient beings, possessing a limbic system with neurological structures and functions similar to those of humans, and thus with the ability to perceive and feel pain, fear, anxiety and pleasure, i.e. emotional states with negative and positive valences. This was established in the protocol on animal welfare in the Amsterdam Treaty (EU, 1997), which was revised and updated in the Lisbon Treaty under the European Commission in 2010 (EC, 2010). By recognising animals as sentient beings, the member states of the European Commission must give full respect to the welfare requirements of certain policies such as those indicated in Article 13 of Title 2, which put animal welfare alongside other principles such as gender equality, guaranteeing social protection, protecting public health, combating discrimination, promoting rural and sustainable development, and protecting personal data (EC, 2007).

Thus, the affective state of animals (feelings or emotions), another dimension of animal welfare, is a key element of quality of life and deserves ethical consideration as an inherent value in the sense of Taylor (2005). However, we know that an animal's quality of life can never be objective. In this regard, ethologist Jeff Rushen (2003) says that it is a mixture of scientific knowledge and value judgements. A high level of welfare requires that the animal experiences comfort, satisfaction and is reasonably free from severe and prolonged pain, fear, hunger and any other state of discomfort, conditions, which can be obtained through the use of alternative systems to total confinement (**Photo 1**) such as organic production systems.

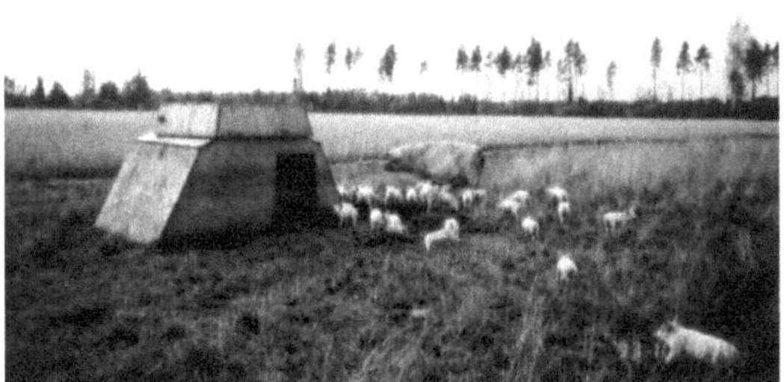

Photo 1. Pigs in a grazing system in Sweden.

On the other hand, according to the animal's inherent nature or naturalness, welfare does not only mean control of pain and suffering, it also encompasses nutrition and the fulfilment of its "genetically encoded nature", what Bernard Rollin (2006) calls *télos*.[19]

Here it is worth digressing and explaining what suffering consists of, given the criticism of intensive animal husbandry by some authors *(e.g.* Mosterín, 1998; Singer, 1999, 2009) as well as **speciesism**"[16][17] , arguing that *"killing is wrong, animals have moral rights, and causing pain and suffering is unacceptable"*. *According* to the expert in the field, Dr. Marian S. Dawkins points out that suffering occurs when unpleasant subjective feelings are intense or continue for a long time, because the animal is unable to carry out the actions that would normally reduce the risk to life and reproduction in those circumstances. Such negative feelings must be avoided, and because they are subjective experiences they are difficult to assess, hence there is little scientific work on the subject. The author describes (Dawkins, 1990) that suffering is a term generally used to refer to adverse physiological and mental states such as pain, fear, frustration, boredom, discomfort, torment or grief, being used as an umbrella term because of the number of mental states it covers. He also warns that it is possible to suffer without pain or to feel pain without suffering, and that the assessment of suffering in animals is difficult, as they cannot communicate directly by means of a common language, and the scientist must therefore rely on careful observations

---

The suffering it entails has inevitably led the public to demand a new ethic (Rollin, 2006. *op. cit.* p. 43).

[17]   Speciesism: Prejudice that consists of taking sides in favour of the interests of one's own species. The term "speciesism" was created by psychologist Richard D. Ryder (1975) in his *Victims of Science: The Use of Animals in Research.* London: Davis-Poynter. 279 pp.; the author applied it to describe the existence of moral discrimination based on animal species difference.

of the animal's behaviour and clinical signs. In later work, he provides an operational definition of suffering, *"as a broad range of unpleasant emotional states"* (Dawkins, 2008).

For his part, Singer (1999, 2009), relying on *emotivist* and *utilitarian theories*, argues that animal suffering is an evil that should be avoided and eradicated as far as possible, and in his work *Animal Liberation, he gives an* exhaustive and critical description of the conditions in which different species are reared in so-called factory farms. Frey (1983), on the other hand, affirms that concern for suffering is compatible with eating meat, and adopts utilitarianism, rejecting Singer's defence of moral vegetarianism as unnecessary.

As can be seen, utilitarianism itself serves to support intensive animal production. According to the Food and Agriculture Organisation of the United Nations (FAO, 2004), consequentialist ethical approaches are the simplest and most obvious way to evaluate an entire system of food and fibre production. The consequentialist understands that what is right, good and proper is determined by the impact of an action or policy on health, wealth and welfare. The intensification prototype aims to increase the total amount of food available without increasing the inputs used. Since food is essential to human life and health, more food has a beneficial effect, especially in the circumstances of food scarcity that have so often characterised human history. Thus, the benefits derived from increased food availability constitute the basic argument for intensification, which is consequentialist in its moral logic.

1.4 Intensive animal production

As already mentioned, domesticated animals used for human consumption are mostly housed in intensive confined housing systems that are highly technical and live in a very different environment from their wild ancestors (Cheeke, 1999; Singer, 1999, 2009). Unfortunately, animal husbandry of yesteryear turned into animal production and exploitation; thus, the old tradition of keeping a limited number of different species on each farm was replaced since the 1950's by keeping only one species and often only one category of animals (Ekesbo, 2010). In this view, less attention was paid to individual animals, and the industry replaced breeding and the values of efficiency and productivity above all else, losing the old contract where producers did well only if the animals were also in favourable conditions (Rollin, 2006).

According to Rollin (2006), there are three major forms of suffering that arise inexorably with intensive livestock farming: the first is *production diseases, i.e.* diseases that are largely the result of the way in which the animal is produced. The second source of suffering is related to the austere, cramped and deprived environmental circumstances in which animals reared in confinement live, while the third form of suffering comes from the sheer size of industrialised farms, which makes it often difficult to detect and treat individual animal problems.

However, it should be noted that these production systems are also characterised by keeping the animals with a minimum of infectious diseases and protected from predators, in addition, they are provided with a feed adequate to their physiological requirements in order to survive and have an optimal production. However, I must emphasise that these systems are the main focus of animal welfare concerns, as it has become evident that they also have their critical points in some management practices (see description by Matheny and Chan, 2005) such as: they suffer from some physical space limitations (Dawkins and Hardie, 1989; Bracke *et al...*, 2002) and social integration with other animals; they are subjected to breeding and genetic programmes aimed at selecting for production traits such as faster growth (Broberg, 2010) through the exogenous use of hormones; they are reared under artificial light cycles; they are subjected to various gadgets and surgical procedures (Stafford and Mellor, 2010) such as de-queening, de-feathering and de-hiving to prevent the display of abnormal behaviours (Lawrence and Rushen, 1993; Vestbjerg Larsen *et al.*, 2016). For example, we often see stereotypical oral behaviours[18] that ungulates display in captivity (**Photo**

2), derived from their foraging behaviour (Bergeron *et al.*, 2006), which, incidentally, are not present in extensive production systems. Also, in pigs housed in intensive production farms with intact tails, outbreaks of tail biting can be observed (Cui *et al.*, 2016; Lahrmann *et al.*, 2016; Wallgren *et al.*, 2016).

The depopulation of laying hens, the dehorning, dehorning and castration of piglets; the disbudding, dehorning and castration of lambs; the dehorning and castration of ruminants, all these practices are generally carried out without the use of anaesthesia or analgesia (except in the European Union) and are

---

central (Mason, G. 2006. Chapter 11. Stereotypic behaviour in captive animals. Fundamentals and implications for welfare and beyond. In: G Mason and J Rushen (eds.), *Stereotypic Animal Behaviour. Fundamentals and Applications for Welfare.* 2nd ed. USA: CABI, pp. 325-356).

therefore referred to by laymen as mutilations. In addition, the principles of ethology, hygiene and comfort of the animals are often not respected, with profitability being the main premise of intensive rearing of domestic species. However, these routine management practices have been changing, and in several countries, as is the case in the European Union (EU Directive 2010/65/EU), the use of analgesic treatments is required by law.

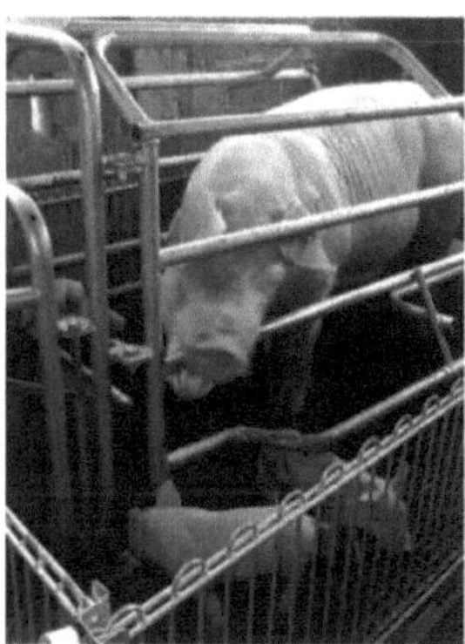

Photo 2. Sow in maternity cages, performing stereotypical bar-biting behaviour.

In several countries, including Mexico, slaughter plants (slaughter is slaughter; slaughter is a religious ritual), slaughter animals must be desensitised prior to slaughter so that they do not suffer and are stunned before they are killed (**Photo 3**). To verify that this happens, an animal welfare assessment and sometimes audit is carried out, which includes several indicators during this process (Grandin, 2007; Gallo and Tadich, 2008; Gregory, 2008; Mota-Rojas *et al.*, 2012). However, it is known that any of the stunning systems currently used represent, to a greater or lesser extent, a stress factor for the animal, which is aggravated by the handling prior to its application (Rosmini, 2010); therefore, killing them with a minimum of stress and pain is a major challenge in *ante-mortem* management practices. In this vein, I would like to point out that the philosopher Jeremy Bentham - the original advocate of sentience as a criterion for moral consideration - admitted that it is perfectly possible to raise animals in comfort and slaughter them painlessly, hence his argument that human consumption of meat is perfectly consistent with an ethic of animal welfare based on sentience

(Callicott, 1998).

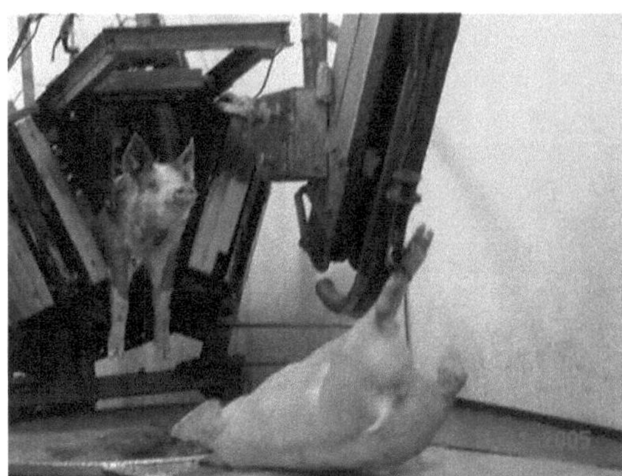

Photo 3. Pigs desensitised by CO_2 in a federal inspection type plant (TIF).
(Courtesy of Dr. Marcelino Becerril j)

On the other hand, fear, stress, malnutrition, uncomfortable environments, lack of disease prevention and treatment, coupled with the absence of allowing normal behaviour such as lying down to rest (**Photo 4**), are factors that affect animal production.

As veterinarians I must point out that we are not unaware that there are potentially unfavourable causes that act to the detriment of the health and welfare of animals, for example pathogens that cause disease, or tissue damage from injuries and trauma acquired in the facilities (Moss, 1992); the expression of negative emotional states such as anxiety, boredom or frustration that come from alterations in internal control and motivation systems (Rollin, 1989; Désire *et al*, 2002; Broom, 2010), or positive emotional states such as pleasure (Balcombe, 2009). We also have the ability to identify suffering through indirect evidence of physical health, clinical signs and behaviour (Dawkins, 1985), along with the manifestations that animals display in the face of pain from pathology or handling (Molony and Kent, 1997; Gregory, 2004; Weary *et al.*, 2006; Dalla Costa *et al*, 2014; Gleerup *et al.*, 2014; McLennan *et al.*, 2014; Rebelo *et al.*, 2014; Stucke *et al.*, 2014; Giminiani *et al.*, 2016) and the stress (Mormede *et al.*, 2007; Palme, 2012; Byrd *et al.*, 2017) that total confinement or fear of humans (Hemsworth *et al.*, 2016; Orlov *et al.*, 2016) causes (see review by Morgan and Tromborg, 2007).

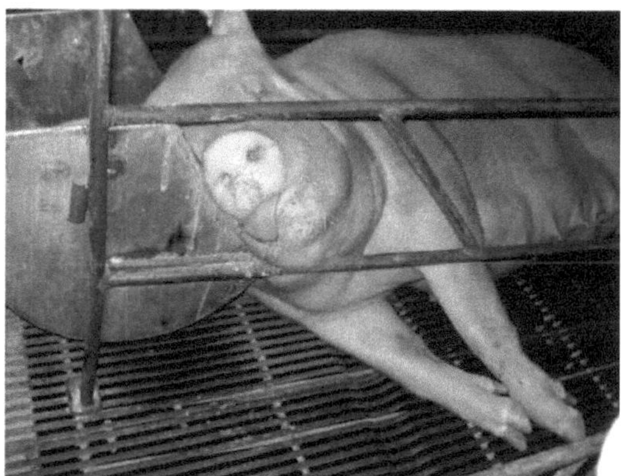

Photo 4. Sow lying in the trough of the maternity pen.

As can be seen, the livestock sector has both positive and negative impacts. Considering animal welfare helps to ensure and enhance the positive impacts and reduce or avoid the negative impacts, and should therefore be a priority everywhere in the world (Appleby, 2017). Animal welfare improves the lives of animals while increasing food safety and meat quality. Likewise, welfare and health are closely related, and in a bidirectional way, since the definition of welfare includes the concept of health and, furthermore, health is defined as *"a state of complete physical, mental and social well-being and not merely the absence of disease or infirmity"* (WHO, 1948). Therefore, we can say that "there is no well-being without health" and that "well-being improves health".

Caring for animal welfare can also help to protect the environment and thus the future sustainability of food production (OIE, 2005).

To conclude this first part, I consider that it is not necessary to rethink identity (whether a non-human animal is a moral agent or not) and the difference with the human being (whether it is sensitive or not to negative emotions), but to focus better on the relationship of responsibility we have towards domestic animals used for human consumption, using scientific criteria of animal welfare. Likewise, we have a moral obligation generated by our emotions towards them as sentient beings, since fortunately, emotions are beginning to cease to be seen as distortions of reason and are now recognised as a determinant of morality. According to Dr Temple Grandin, *"our relationship with livestock should be symbiotic; symbiosis is a biological concept that explains a mutually beneficial relationship between two different species. "Killing animals to produce food is ethical as long as the animals have a 'life worth living'"* (Grandin, 2014). This position is consistent with Mellor's (2016) view described above.

2. The habit of eating meat

Animal welfare science and especially ethology - the science of animal behaviour - start from a very solid theoretical framework, based on the four classic questions of the ethologist and Nobel Prize winner Nikolaas Tinbergen (1963): cause, ontogeny, phylogeny and adaptation.

Behaviours, according to Tinbergen (1963), can be understood in four different ways in terms of their causes: ***phylogenic causes****, which* tell us when did the behaviour emerge in the evolutionary history of the species? This clearly refers to questions of an evolutionary nature, and as the behaviour does not leave fossils, it requires comparative studies of closely related living species in order to explain it. ***Ontogenetic causes*** require an analysis of the questions: how does behaviour change over the course of a subject's life, how does the environment influence it, what maturation and learning processes are important? While ***proximate or immediate causes*** tell us how do they occur, what are the mechanisms that control behaviour and how do they act, what are the internal and external stimuli that produce behaviour? And finally, the ***ultimate or remote causes*** indicate what the behaviour is for or what are the selective pressures to which the behaviour responds; they are a category about the adaptive significance of the behaviour and indicate why the behaviours occur, what is their function, adaptation or adaptive advantage? Contextualised in ethical theories, the latter would correspond to ***deontological theories***[22] , which attempt to answer what we are obliged to do.

Proximate cause (mechanism) and ontogeny are proximate mechanisms, explaining **how** behaviour occurs in the particular individual. Phylogeny and ultimate cause or function (survival value) are ultimate mechanisms and explain **why** behaviour appears in the species. All causes are equally important, i.e. we cannot claim to understand a phenomenon until we have answered all four questions.

According to some critics, today's ethical vegetarians recognise that humans are predatory animals (though not carnivores, at least omnivores) and that meat is a natural constituent of the human diet. But if eating meat is natural for humans, how can it be wrong (Fink, 2011)? Moreover, appealing to the ***predation argument****, according* to Kent Baldner (1990), *"if killing for food is morally*

---

[22] Deontological theories: from the Greek *deontos,* meaning "necessity" or "obligation". Ethical theories that emphasise right and wrong or obligation (Rollin, BE. 2006. *op. cit.* p. 23.).

justifiable for natural predators, it would have to be morally justifiable for human predators as well, whether 'individual hunters or corporate factory farms'". According to philosopher Cora Diamond (1978), "we do *not eat them because we do not consider them food for man. If we didn't consider them good to eat, we wouldn't consider them food, and vice versa; we eat animals because we consider them food".* Next, in this second part of the essay, I propose to analyse and justify meat-eating behaviour by addressing Tinbergen's four questions, starting with the evolutionary ones.

2.1 The phylogenic causes of meat eating

How has behaviour evolved in the species? Nowadays, evolution is called phylogeny, the study of the phylogenetic history of that behaviour, of its precursors, which leads to understanding why the behaviour has the current form and not another.

The encephalisation of man

Humans have lived a hunter-gatherer life for most of their existence, from their appearance some 100,000 years ago until about 10,000 years ago, when a cultural and demographic revolution of great significance, agriculture and livestock farming, began to spread around the world (Viejo Montesinos, 1996). Our primitive ancestors, the australopithecines, consumed carrion left by the large predators of the time. Even today, one of the preferred foods of the Hadza, a hunter-gatherer human population in Tanzania, is carrion (Vinyes, 2005). Blumenschine and Cavallo (1992) point out that "*the consumption of meat by early hominids helped shape the evolution of the brain, behaviour and the ability to create tools",* highlighting the importance of meat consumption in the evolutionary development of our genus.

To better understand the process of encephalisation, let us review the cranial capacity of some hominids[23] , according to the theologian and molecular geneticist, Francisco J. Ayala (2011). The first hominid fossil was found in 1889 on the island of Java, it belonged to a bipedal man *(Homo erectus)* who lived from about 1.8 million years ago until approximately 400,000 years ago, the capacity of his small skull was 850 to 1,100 cm^3 (it could hold a brain weighing less than a kilo; 1 kg is 1,000 grams, equivalent to 454 cm^3); as a reference, the

---

[23] The primates that were ancestors of man, after our lineage separated from the chimpanzee, are called hominids (Ayala, FJ. 2011. *¿Soy un Mono?*, Barcelona: Ariel, p. 20.).

skull of a modern human is about 1,300 cm^3 . Hominids classified as *Homo habilis* (lived in tropical Africa 1.5 to 2.5 million years ago) were the first to make the simplest stone tools, had a cranial capacity of about 600 cm^3 , larger than that of early hominids, but less than half the size of a modern human brain. *Homo erectus* made more advanced tools than *Homo habilis* and were the first intercontinental nomads. Homo *erectus was* followed by *Homo neanderthalis* and *Homo sapiens*, our species (**Photo 5**).

Palaeontological findings at Olduvai Gorge, Tanzania by archaeologist Manuel Domínguez-Rodrigo and his team confirm that *Homo erectus* consumed meat. It is the archaeological site containing the largest number of hominin bones and sacrificed animals from the Pleistocene (Domínguez-Rodrigo *et al.*, 2013).

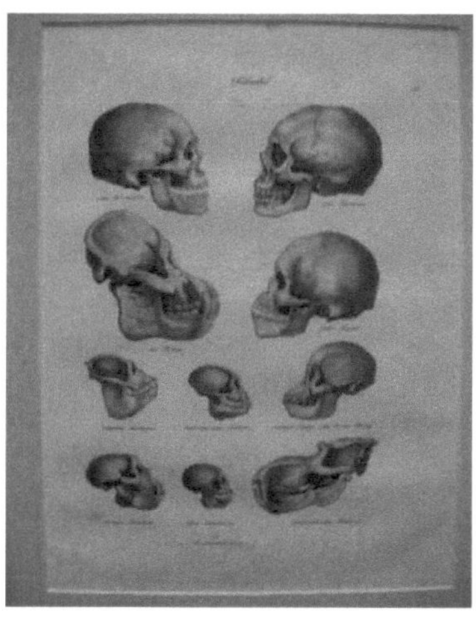

Photo 5. Cranial capacity of different hominid species.

According to researchers Aiello and Wheeler (1995), individuals with relatively large brains would have the minimum intelligence to be the first to make tools with which to break the shafts of bones in order to gain access to the marrow, where the most energetic nutrients are found. Thus, a diet rich in animal fats and proteins would allow a progressive increase in brain volume, and thus a progressive development of intelligence. According to this hypothesis, the consumption of large quantities of meat meant that large brains made it possible to have a minimum of intelligence to be able to manufacture the tools that made it possible to butcher and dismember the remains of large animals. The basic assumption of this premise is based on the assumption that large brains are obtained after consuming meat, an assumption that Marmelada (2007) also makes. Likewise, anthropologist Craig Stanford (1999) believes that the sharing of meat set in motion the evolution of the brain by facilitating social intelligence. By becoming omnivores, the genus *Homo* was able to adapt to almost every ecosystem on the planet, reaching and colonising it over time.

Biologist Colin Tudge, for his part, stresses that the palentological evidence suggests that human hunters, not the climate, as was once assumed, wiped out the huge fauna that existed in the Americas and Australia. If climate had been responsible, it is presumed that the smaller animals would have suffered even more than the larger ones; however, they remained without considerable damage. It can be reasonably assumed, according to Tudge (2000), that the large herbivores became extinct because they became a target for hunters, and the large predators disappeared because their basic prey died out. However, this hypothesis has not yet been tested.

It is worth noting that 2.5 million years ago our hominid ancestors ate more meat than today's chimpanzees do. Today's adult chimpanzees hunt rats, squirrels, small antelopes, baboons and even baby chimpanzees, but their favourite delicacy is a monkey called the red colobus (**Fig. 1**). However, meat accounts for only 3 to 4% of their usual diet, and the most voracious carnivorous chimpanzees eat no more than 50 grams per day (Stanford *et al.*, 1994).

Figure 1. Chimpanzee meat consumption preferences.

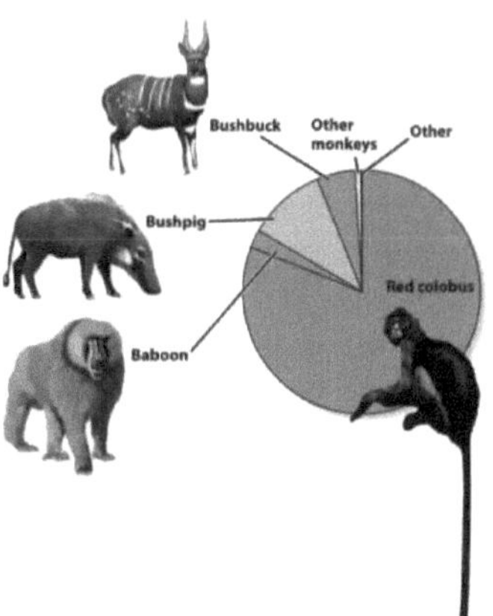

Fuente: Stanford (1995).

The domestication of animals

In the last 11,000 years some peoples engaged in food production, i.e. the domestication[24] of wild animals and the cultivation of plants, as well as the consumption of livestock and the resulting crops, which indirectly constituted, in the synthesis of anthropologist Jared Diamond, *"a prerequisite for the development of firearms, germs and steel".* Diamod (1998) reveals that the species that man managed to domesticate have been almost exclusively Eurasian. The surprisingly small number of domesticated mammals, 14, of which only five became widespread and important worldwide: the cow, the sheep, the goat, the pig and the horse. More specifically, of the 148 large candidate species to be domesticated, i.e. herbivorous or omnivorous terrestrial wild mammals with an average weight of 45 kg, only 14, i.e. 21%, were domesticated (Diamond, 1998). One of the reasons was due to poor biomass conversion efficiency, which is in the order of 10%, as will be discussed in the last chapter.

Domestication involves the transformation of the wild animal into something more

---

[24] Domestication: The process by which animals come to live in a state of true symbiosis with humans. In a state of domesticity, animals depend on man for their livelihood, reproduce under his direction and in turn, in most cases, are useful and productive (Oteyza, J. and Carmona, JR. 1985. *op. cit.* p. 82). For Price and King, domestication is an evolutionary process that involves genotypic adaptation of animals to the captive environment (Price, EO. and King, JA. 1973. Domestication and adaptation. In: ESE Hafez (ed.), *Adaptation of Domestic Animals.* Spain, Barcelona: Ed. Labor, pp. 53-69).

useful to humans, through the control of reproduction and food supply. It has been postulated that domesticated animals have lost many of the biological adaptive characteristics of their wild ancestors. Several domestic animal species have smaller brains and less developed sensory organs than their wild ancestors because they no longer need the large brains and more developed sensory organs that their ancestors relied on to escape from wild predators (Ginzburg, 1996; Diamond, 1998). Zoologist Helmut Hemmer (1990), points out that domestic animals have a lower *"environmental appreciation'* than wild animals, their alertness and fear responses, and their motor activity is lower, i.e. they have less need to rely on their "wits" to survive and can relax their guard under human care. However, this does not detract from the fact that, in the light of scientific evidence, they are sentient and conscious beings as reviewed in the first chapter.

Also science writer Stephen Budiansky (quoted by Tudge, 2000), argues that animals that lent themselves to domestication obtained protection and food, and were therefore able to raise their offspring in better conditions than those that continued in the wild. To a large extent, an animal's suitability for domestication is under genetic control. Because several species in the wild have become extinct or are in danger of extinction, domesticated cattle are very numerous today thanks to domestication. Budiansky (1992) concludes that domestication can be considered not as dominance, but as an evolutionary strategy, a win-win pact, beneficial for both humans and animals. However, as the philosopher Martha Nussbaum (2007) points out, the asymmetry of power between humans and animals is too great for us to imagine a genuine contract with them. Although animals cannot make contracts with us, even if we would like them to (Narveson, 1983), and although they are not members of the moral community, this does not mean that their treatment is irrelevant, especially if their protection and care depend on us.

2.2 Ontogenetic causes of meat eating

Ontogeny is development, so how does behaviour change over the course of an individual's life?

Consumption, society and culture

The evolution of food throughout history has been influenced by social, racial, political and economic changes (Harris, 1980; Castillo and Leon, 2002; Hill and York, 2003). In addition, it is governed by the system of beliefs and values existing in any culture[25] and time, which may in turn determine which foods are accepted or rejected in each situation and for each type of person (Contreras, 2007), with meat being the food on which most cultural and religious prohibitions regulate its consumption *(e.g.* pork among Muslims and Jews; beef among Hindus) (Rozin *et al.,* 2000). However, it is worth noting that people in India, despite not eating beef - a constitutionally forbidden habit in that country (Chigateri, 2011) - happily consume as much milk, butter, cheese and yoghurt as they can afford, with ghee - diluted butter - being the preferred cooking fat in traditional cuisine. For their part, Buddhists may not slaughter or witness the slaughter of animals, but they may eat meat as long as they do not personally terminate the animal's life; thus, for example, Thai Buddhists consume significant amounts of pork, buffalo meat, beef, chicken, duck, silkworms, snails, shrimp and crabs (Harris, 2010).

During the Middle Ages in Europe, meat was consumed in excess because of relatively low population density and extensive green pastures. With population growth, fresh meat became a luxury item until the advent of industrialisation from the 19th century onwards multiplied productivity and made the final product cheaper.

People depend on animals not only for income, food and clothing, but also for social status, security, comfort, social contact and cultural identification (Foresight The Future of Food and Farming, 2011; Appleby, 2015). For example, for 90% of the world's rural landowners - nearly one billion people - animals are their primary income (Appleby, 2015). Historically, in most Western societies, meat consumption has represented social and economic prestige; as countries improve their economies, meat consumption increases. In the second half of the 20th century, meat production increased fivefold, with *per capita* consumption more than doubling. This has meant that livestock production has taken up most of the arable land. Since 1960, *per capita* meat consumption has increased six-fold in Japan and fifteen-fold in China (Halweil and Nieremberg, 2008).

On the other hand, the current human population exceeds 6 billion, with about 1 billion pigs, 1.3 billion cows, 1.8 billion sheep and goats, and 15.4 billion chickens. This growth is due to the fact that more developing countries with growing economies are willing to consume more and more meat (Gold, 2004).

---

[25] Anthropologist Mervin Harris defines culture as the adaptive capacity of human beings and their main weapon for survival. (Harris, M. 1980. *Cows, Pigs, Wars and Witches: The Enigmas of Culture.* Madrid: Alianza Editorial, 246 pp.).

According to data from the Food and Agriculture Organisation of the United Nations (FAO), by 2050 more than half of the population will belong to the middle class, which will generate a 60% increase in the demand for animal-based food (FAO, 2017). In Mexico, for example, five out of every 10 pesos are spent on the purchase of animal products, which represents 75% of the food energy supply (Notimex, 2014).

Singer (1999) postulates in his utilitarian ethics the **principle of equal consideration of interests**[25] , which considers the ethical aspect of the use of meat for human food, and states that a relatively secondary human interest must be weighed against the life and welfare of the animals concerned. Singer (1979) argues that killing an animal for food is not an ethical problem if the animal had a pleasurable life and after killing it is replaced by another animal that also has a pleasurable life and would not exist if the first animal had not been killed. However, it must be taken into account that the value of each individual's preference to continue living is immeasurable, according to de Lora (2003). Moreover, the principle of equal consideration of interests does not allow for the sacrifice of primary interests over secondary ones; the strongest interest must prevail no matter who has it, which is why Singer (1979, 1989) argues that [26]

that we should all be vegetarians. Mark Rowlands (1998), in turn, also argues that raising and killing nonhuman animals for food is morally wrong, because no one would choose the existence of such a possibility under the *veil of ignorance*[27] [28] .

According to J. Baird Callicott (1998), a leading philosopher of an **ecocentrist environmental ethic**[23] , the economy of nature is constituted by a system of

---

[26] Principle of equal consideration of interests: According to Peter Singer, *"the essence of this principle is that in our moral deliberations we give equal weight to the similar interests of all those who are affected by our actions. It implies that our concern for others should not depend on what they are like, what capacities they possess, even if the characteristics of those affected by our actions vary precisely what we do as a consequence of this concern"* (Singer, P. 2009. *Practical Ethics.* Madrid: Akal, pp. 32, 66).

[27] The veil of ignorance is a concept used by the philosopher John Rawls to arrive at the two principles of his theory of social justice. The veil of ignorance is that when people choose the principles of justice they do not know what their specific circumstances (what social position they will occupy) will be. Since the principles that will emerge are not designed to the advantage or disadvantage of individuals in a particular scenario, the principles that emerge from the veil of ignorance can be considered just (Caballero, JF. 2006. John Rawls' theory of justice. *Voices and Contexts,* 2 (1): 1-22).

[28] Ethics based on a sense of community between humans and all living things, morally condemns human actions in terms of their environmental impact (Callicott, JB. 1998. In search of an environmental ethic. In: Kwiatkowska, T. and Issa, J. (eds.), *The Pathways of Environmental Ethics. An Anthology of Contemporary Texts.* Mexico: CONACyT, UAM, Plaza y Valdés, pp. 85-159).

trophic relationships where energy (the circulant of the natural economy) only flows through the ecosystem when one being eats another. Callicott (1998) writes: *"Sudden, premature and often painful deaths are fundamental and unappealable ecological facts of life. A system purged of pain - what seems to be a moral ideal according to the theory of animal liberation advocate Peter Singer - would be both enormously impoverished and critically lacking in stability".* He thus disqualifies Singer's (1998) utilitarian ethics because, according to Callicot, it does not provide any theoretical means of ethically distinguishing between wild and domestic animals. Similarly, for the philosopher Oscar Horta (2012), the suffering and death in nature is considerably greater than it would be in a situation of stability, because it implies that numerous animals have to die on a massive scale (from starvation, devoured by other animals, or for other reasons) when a certain population of animals dwindles.

Tom Regan (1999), considered the pioneering philosophical leader of the animal rights movement, defends the intrinsic moral value of animals and their right to live in the best possible conditions. In this way, he advocates the abolition of all human practices aimed at causing suffering or humiliation to any animal. Regan takes an **abolitionist** stance[29] to any human use of animals, including food production. In this regard, although it is true that in some farmers the **Cartesian thinking** prevails[30] that animals are mere machines that do not feel, and some cruelty still prevails in some systems, this concern has led to more awareness in the schools and faculties of MVZ in the country among students and researchers, so that the subject of animal welfare has been incorporated into the *curriculum* of most universities (Aluja, 2011; Alonso-Spilsbury *et al.,* 2012b; Galindo, 2012; Mota-Rojas *et al.,* 2018) with a view to conducting welfare assessments of animals on different farms and stables, with the purpose of providing recommendations to owners to improve the living conditions of food animals under their care, while students acquire professional competencies in their

---

[29] Abolitionism: An emerging radical movement that addresses the rights of nonhuman animals. The movement calls for a complete cessation in the use of animals through the abolition of non-human animal ownership status and the adoption of veganism and non-violence (Wrenn, C. 2012. Abolitionist animal rights: critical comparisons and challenges within the animal rights movement. *Interface,* 4 (2): 438-458).

[30] Cartesian thought: More than 300 years ago, the French philosopher, mathematician and scientist, René Descartes argued that *"animals are pure automatons which, by virtue of their lack of soul and reason, do not even have sensations, and that it is we men who interpret their movements as if they were sensations"* (Descartes, R. 1988. *Discourse on Method.* Madrid: Austral. Tr. by Manuel García Morente, 83 pp.).

training.

Ervin Laszlow (2001) - a philosopher of science - notes that global meat consumption increased from 40 million tonnes in 1950 to 196 million tonnes in 1999. According to current projections, the world's population may reach approximately 9.7 billion by 2050 (FAO, 2017), of which many will continue to consume meat. On the assumption that it would ever be decided not to exploit domestic animals and to keep them in free-range conditions in the open air simply because they are beings that possess a value in themselves, which does not depend on the opinion of others, i.e. they have inherent worth as Regan (1983) points out, or because, as Singer (1998) argues, intensive animal husbandry violates the principle of equality of interests, I wonder if they - the advocates of this position - have ever thought about what would happen to those billions of animals mentioned a few paragraphs ago, where would be the land capacity to keep them free?, Who would look after their health, especially with so many catastrophes caused by climate change, or what would happen to natural resources in terms of the pollution they generate, which I will discuss in the last section. The answer, in my opinion, is that from a biocentrist or abolitionist point of view, it would not be sustainable or ethical to keep all these animals until they die for natural reasons - assuming that in the environment where they are released there are no more carnivores to prey on them - their longevity would simply not allow it! Consider that a calf can live for 25 to 30 years; they are killed at one to two years; the pig, which would live to 15 years, is killed at 6 months of age; the sheep would also live to 15 years but is killed at 3 to 10 months; and the chicken, which would live to 10 years, grows and fattens very quickly, being killed at only 6 weeks of age.

Although death constitutes the imputation of a harm because it represents the deprivation of positive things in a being, and the harm of death affects the enjoyment of life (Horta, 2012, personal com. personal in a conference given at UAM-X), based on classical utilitarianism, I consider that it would be convenient to continue raising animals under more "friendly" systems and with animal welfare criteria, that is, to continue killing farm animals under our care, in order to keep them alive in a certain period of time that implies the commercial production cycles for each species as we know them in the area of animal production, described in the previous paragraph. From this perspective, I would be appealing to the *logic of the larder*[3] , by the moralist writer Sir Leslie Stephen (1896) - the father of

[31] According to Leslie Stephen, an intellectual of the Victorian aristocracy, we do animals a favour by buying meat, eggs and milk, for if we did not buy these products, few animals could exist (Stephen, L. 1896. *Social Rights and Duties: Addresses to Ethical Societies.* NY: Macmillan & Co.). The *"logic of the larder"* results from the common notion that the supply of farm animals more or less follows the demand for their products, and the less common notion that the world is much better off if it has more animals in existence. This argument is now defended by a number of thinkers, including ethologists Mike Appleby - Virginia Woolf - for one of their premises is that killing animals is morally permissible and even obligatory, as long as the animals have pleasurable lives. In this respect, Visac (2013) notes, *"by doing so, one maximises welfare by killing animals that exist only for that purpose".* This argument is like the paradox of natural parks or management units for wildlife conservation where the management of animals becomes difficult and some have to be sacrificed to maintain the ecological balance, or even hunting permits are granted, even though these animals have the right to life, which makes it possible to conserve more specimens in these units with the financial resources obtained, thus achieving sustainable use. I also agree with Frey (1983), who argues that the disappearance of meat consumption would cause problems and questions whether the utility achieved by its disappearance would be more harmful than beneficial in the long run.

It is worth mentioning that one of the great detractors of the *logic of the pantry* was Henry S. Salt (1914), vegetarian, pacifist and opponent of vivisection, pioneer of animal rights. On the other hand, Bart Gruzalski (1989; quoted by de Lora, 2003), states that being vegetarian, from a utilitarian point of view, besides being absurd, can be counterproductive, he argues, it could happen that the effect of marginal vegetarianism lowers meat prices with the consequent reaction of producers in terms of making production more intensive and thus, following the thinking of several vegetarians, causing more animal suffering.

An alternative to the excessive meat consumption that occurs in some northern hemisphere countries is reduction. It is estimated that a 10% reduction in consumption would allow 11 million more tonnes of grain to be available for human consumption and this grain could be used to feed all the human beings who die of hunger every year (**Photo 6**), estimated at some 60 million people (Laszlow, 2001); although the problem of hunger, as we know, depends not only on the availability of food, but also on its more equitable distribution.

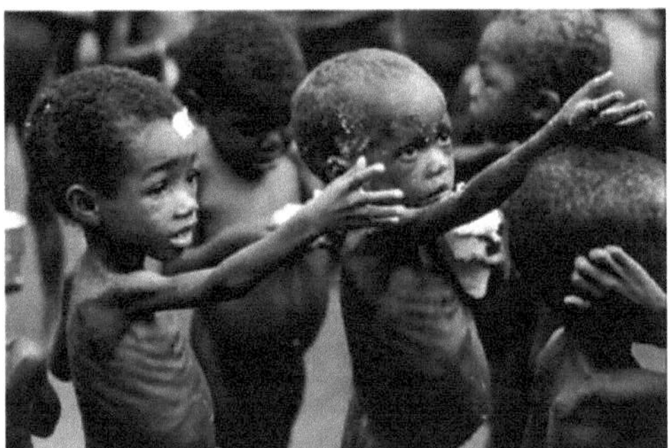

Photo 6. Caquéxic children begging for food.

2.3 The proximate causes of eating meat

Physiological mechanism

Proximate causes in Tinbergen's strict sense refer to the study of the mechanisms of behavioural control or motivation, what are the internal and external stimuli that trigger behaviour? For the case at hand, feeding behaviour is a central nervous system-mediated process involving the intake of food, water and electrolytes. The hypothalamus and its hunger (medial hypothalamic nuclei; Margules and Olds, 1962) and satiety (ventromedial hypothalamic nucleus; Ehrlich, 1964) centres are involved, along with a network of circuits that regulate intake and ingestion that make connections with the cerebral cortex, implying learning of the feeding process and the importance of cognitive aspects. Hormonal, metabolic and neural signals are involved in its regulation.

The well-known stimulant effect of meat is due to its hypoxanthine content, a stimulant produced in the muscle fibres as a result of the degradation processes that take place in the carcass after the animal is slaughtered (Vinyes, 2010). Eating meat is also pleasurable for its texture, because of the particular work done by our teeth when we chew it. In addition, it is known that high-fat foods have the power to modify the motivation and reward systems in the brain; certain neuropeptides are activated during activities involving reward and pleasure (Choi *et al.,* 2009).

Likewise, aroma and flavour are sensory properties of great importance for the meat consumer, since in combination with colour and texture, they determine the quality, acceptance or rejection of meat and meat products. The aroma and flavour of meat are generated after heat treatment, as raw meat has a metallic taste similar to blood. Cooked meat, on the other hand, produces a large quantity of volatile and non-volatile compounds that impart the aroma and flavour of cooked meat (Ponce, 2010a).

However, the factor that most influences whether we find a food delicious or disgusting is culture. Daniel Fessler, an evolutionary anthropologist, has studied food taboos in 78 human societies. Together with one of his students (Fessler and Navarrete, 2003), he found that perfectly edible meats were six times more likely to be forbidden than vegetables, fruits or grains. Paul Rozin and his colleagues (Rozin *et al.,* 2000) found that eating meat is more repugnant to people who are vegetarians for moral reasons than to those who are vegetarians for health reasons. While for anthropologist Marvin Harris (2010), dietary preferences and aversions arise from favourable practical cost-benefit ratios.

When considering a food as necessary for our growth and health, it is not enough to take into account only its nutritional impact on our organism (analysing the benefits of minerals, vitamins, nutrients, etc.), but we must also not forget the cultural meaning it represents and how it affects our psychological dimension and our consequent state of health (Moyano, 2018). What we eat can affect our mood, a dimension of human well-being (Challam, 2007).

Seneca warned that among the great meat eaters we could find tyrants, organisers of massacres, instigators of wars and murders, and slave traders, while those fed on the fruits of the earth tended to be gentler and more peaceful in character. In this regard, an ethnobotany student, Andrew Gerren (2012), conducted a survey of vegetarian and omnivore students, finding inconsistent results regarding the subjective well-being of vegetarians, possibly attributed to the fact that some vegetarians chose this lifestyle for ethical reasons such as guilt about killing animals, which led to an increase in the well-being of these participants. In that study, a high percentage of vegetarians reported regular marijuana use, which may have led to depression caused by chemical imbalances in the brain. In contrast, Michalak *et al.* (2012) observed mental disorders such as anxiety in vegetarians, when compared to those who ate an omnivorous diet. It is striking that the authors found no evidence for a causal role of vegetarian diet in the aetiology of mental disorders, rather their results suggest that the presentation of a mental disorder increases the likelihood of choosing to be vegetarian, which leads us to think that psychological factors influence both positions, i.e. the likelihood of deciding to be vegetarian or not and the likelihood of developing a mental disorder. However, there is no conclusive data in this area.

2.4 The ultimate causes of eating meat

Ultimate causes refer to the function, adaptation or adaptive advantage of the behaviour: how does the behaviour contribute to survival and reproductive success, how does the behaviour increase the biological efficiency of the individual displaying it? Recall that ultimate causes act on the species.

Nutritional value

With regard to the attitude held by those who consider that there is no reason to justify the killing of animals, arguing that: *"humans can live without eating animal protein", I* supplement my objection with the following scientific reasoning.

Meat is an integral part of the human diet (Young *et al.,* 2013). The moment we switched from a predominantly plant-based diet to a more carnivorous diet, we became dependent on animal protein as a source of vitamin B12, among other nutrients. Like everything in evolution, it is a matter of cost-benefit. We gained access to a denser nutritional source, which allowed us to shorten our digestive system and divert this energy to our great consumer, the brain. The caecum, an area of the large intestine that in many herbivores *(e.g.* rabbits and horses) is enlarged, is vestigial in humans like the appendix. In short, humans are food opportunists who basically eat any edible plant or animal, with a diet preferably low in fibre (Cheeke, 1999).

The importance of meat is very relevant today, as a lack of meat - and vitamin B12 - can lead to serious problems, especially in the brain and nervous system, such as fatigue, clinical depression, or poor memory. And in children it can cause difficulties in the growth of both the body and the brain itself, perennial problems that arise during the growth phase rather than in adulthood when the body is already formed (Craig, 2010).

Nowadays, meat is a common source of proteins, fats and minerals in the human diet, and is the most highly valued and appreciated in the markets because it provides the diet with the essential amino acids that the human organism is not capable of synthesising on its own; it provides the amino acids essential for the following processes: tissue maintenance, repair and growth; production of plasma proteins and muscle creatinine; synthesis of enzymes, hormones, polypeptides and some neurotransmitters; formation of hair, skin and nails; and synthesis of milk proteins. In addition, essential amino acids and bioactive compounds are important in the prevention of sarcopenia and in maintaining the functional intestinal environment, via meat-derived nucleotides and nucleosides (Young *et al.*, 2013).

Clinical nutrition researcher Loren Cordain and his team (Cordain *et al.*, 2001), after examining the diets of hundreds of hunter-gatherer groups, found that these groups obtained, on average, two-thirds of their calories from animal meat. They found no hunter-gatherer society surviving on a diet containing less than 15% animal products.

As far as true digestibility is concerned, proteins of animal origin (eggs, milk, fish and meat) have values of around 95%, while those of vegetable origin commonly included in our diets are much lower (FAO/WHO/UNU, 1991). These lower digestibility values are due to the nature of the protein itself and also to dietary factors that modify its absorption, such as fibre, tannins and protein enzyme inhibitors, as would be the case of the trypsin inhibitor present in soya. Moreover, according to FAO (1991), animal proteins have a very adequate pattern of essential amino acids, even exceeding the values of an ideal protein. In contrast, vegetable proteins, with the exception of soya protein, do not meet human protein needs, as they are deficient in at least one or two essential amino acids. To explain the importance of the quality and quantity of amino acids in the human diet, just one example: wheat contains all the essential amino acids, but in order to obtain sufficient quantities of the scarcest ones, a man weighing 80 kilos would have to gorge himself daily on
1.5 kg of wholemeal bread. To achieve the same level of protein security, you would only need 340 grams of meat (Harris, 2010).

On the other hand, meat consumption is criticised for its cholesterol content. Cholesterol is a precursor substance for the production of bile acids in the human body; these compounds are necessary for the proper absorption of fats during the process of food intake (Braverman, 1994). Cholesterol also helps in the production of hormones involved in the regulation of sodium and potassium storage (the hormone aldosterone) in the human body; It is also necessary for the production of oestrogen, testosterone and progesterone - sex hormones - necessary for the normal development of the human body to reach sexual maturity.

Also, vitamins D2 and D3 are formed from cholesterol and other nutrients present in the human body (Swenson and Reece, 1993; Braverman, 1994). Certainly, growth and the onset of puberty in vegetarian children is not as rapid compared to meat eaters (Vinyes, 2005).

Health

While it is true that vegetarians are known for being healthy, there are controversies about diets. Let us first review the concept of vegetarianism. The word "vegetarian" comes from the Latin *"vegetus", an* adjective meaning "whole, healthy, fresh or vigorous", as in *"Homo vegetus",* a mentally and physically vigorous, healthy, alert, full of life and activity; the original meaning of the word implies a balanced philosophy and moral sense of life, much more than a diet of fruits and vegetables. Most people who are considered vegetarians also tend to eat some animal products, such as honey, dairy products and eggs (ovo-lacto-vegetarian diet). Those who eat only plant-based foods are called *"vegetarians", and "vegans" are those* who do not use any animal products in their daily lives (clothes, shoes, food, etc.) (Vinyes, 2005), i.e. they are true vegetarians (Harris, 2010). Ethical vegetarianism begins with the recognition that other creatures feel and that their feelings are similar to ours; ethical vegetarianism is practised by people whose eating habits demonstrate ethical and moral respect for animals by refusing to eat meat and animal products.

In a study, Herrmann *et al.* (2003) found that in 174 apparently healthy individuals in Germany and the Netherlands, 92% of those following a strict vegan diet were deficient in vitamin B12. Among ovo-lacto-vegetarians 2 out of 3, and only 5% of those consuming animal protein, were deficient. Thus, vegetarian diets have been found to be deficient in several nutrients including: protein, iron, zinc, calcium, vitamin B12 and A, n-3 fatty acids and iodine. Most deficiencies are due to poor dietary planning, as shown by numerous studies *(e.g.* Leitzmann, 2005). However, according to the American Dietetic Association (American Dietetic Association, 2009), a well-balanced vegetarian diet is suitable for all ages and physiological states, from childhood to adulthood, in pregnant women and athletes, which reduces various health risks such as: cardiovascular diseases, hypertension, type 2 diabetes, cancer, osteoporosis, dementia, gallstones, rheumatoid arthritis, stroke, cataracts, Alzheimer's disease, as well as a decrease in age-associated functions (Liu, 2003; Leitzmann, 2005). However, in a meta-analysis involving the integration of five retrospective studies with a total of 76,172 people, it was found that there was no significant difference in mortality between vegetarians and non-vegetarians from cerebrovascular disease, stomach, colorectal, lung, breast and prostate cancer, or all causes combined (Key *et al.,* 1999).

Quantitatively and qualitatively, animal-based foods remain a better source of protein than plant-based foods (Harris, 2010). An alternative to counterbalance the disadvantages brought about by deficiencies due to a lack of meat consumption is to practice what is currently known as *flexitarianism, an* adjective given to those who occasionally eat meat (Flail, 2011; Raphaely and Marinova, 2014ab). In the end, let us remember that, as Dr. Hector Bourges points out, no single food contains all the nutrients necessary for good health, and no single food is responsible for causing disease (Bourges, 1982, 1984).

The controversy over which diet is better will continue, as there is no consensus among proponents and/or detractors. It must be admitted that excesses are harmful, especially in the *fast food* diet consumed by people in developed countries, which is increasingly hypercaloric. This is not the case in some developing nations, such as several African countries, where nutritional deficiencies are common and where the incorporation of meat and milk would mean substantial improvements in the health of the population (Walker *et al.,* 2005), as well as in our country, where a close relationship has been observed between the ingestion of animal-based foods and the improvement of physical and cognitive development in children (Allen *et al.,* 1992). Given such scenarios, the World Health Organisation estimates that while undernutrition is falling globally, almost 11% of the population still goes to bed hungry, and micronutrient deficiencies affect more than two billion people (FAO, 2017), causing half of all child deaths in developing countries. The main foods - blends of fortified maize or wheat and soy flours - do not meet the minimum nutritional needs of the most vulnerable children aged 6-24 months (WHO, 1996, 2000).

Article 25 of the Universal Declaration of Human Rights (UDHR, 1948) states that everyone has the right to food, and being well fed is, from the ethical perspective invoked by the Nobel Prize winner in economics, Amarthya Sen (1993), decisive for being free. In this regard, the philosopher John Rawls (2011), based on his **theory of social justice**[31] , which consists of recommending the option that is

---

[31] In 1971, John Rawls published his work "A Theory of Justice". Broadly speaking, Rawls' theory considers that the principles of justice that are the subject of an agreement between rational, free and equal persons in a fair contractual situation can have universal and unconditional validity (Caballero, JF. 2006. *op. cit.*).

expected to have the greatest value for the group with the least economic resources and the most vulnerable in society, makes it possible to formulate ethical justifications that favour the interests of poor or marginalised people over those who are better off. He points out that while it would be highly desirable to increase the consumption of animal products in developing countries to combat malnutrition, its implementation would not necessarily be successful.

3. Environmental ethics and sustainability in meat production

The intensification of the livestock sector means more food for growing populations, but there are also a number of ethical issues related to the use of resources in the livestock sector, food safety and quality, fairness and treatment of animals, and contamination of land, water and air. There are also direct issues associated with disease transmission and general food safety (FAO, 2004).

Teresa Kwiatkowska (2008) - a contemporary environmental philosopher - stresses that any worthwhile **environmental ethic**[32] has an obligation not only to animals, plants, species and ecosystems, but also to humans in their specifically human environment, and to their commercial and political interests to provide crucial information for ethical decision-making. This is undoubtedly a contentious issue as the continued expansion of agricultural production must be balanced against the costs of ongoing environmental degradation.

The lines of dependency for food and other services are known as food or trophic chains. For Aldo Leopold (1963), forester, ecologist and environmentalist, founder of the **Earth ethic**[33] , the soil-oak-oak-deer-Indian chain has now become soil-corn-cow-farmer. The rapid growth of livestock farming is causing changes in agricultural land use with considerable effects on the environment. In Latin America, drivers of climate change include mainly forest clearing and cattle and soy production, with social costs resulting from deforestation and the consequences in terms of soil degradation and erosion, water pollution, loss of biodiversity and loss of carbon contributing to global warming (FAO, 2013, 2017). It is estimated that every year, around 0.3% to 0.4% of forest land in the area is converted to livestock (FAO, 2009). For example, the Amazon rainforest is being destroyed at a rate of 25,000 km^2 per year, i.e. 4.5 hectares of forest are deforested every minute (Camacho, 2004). This problem contributes to habitat destruction and is a threat to biodiversity.

The Organisation for Economic Co-operation and Development and the Food and Agriculture Organisation of the United Nations (FAO) estimate that to meet

---

[32] One of its core positions holds that the basis of our moral obligations to the natural world (plants, animals, ecosystems and sometimes inanimate objects) lies in its importance for the physical, intellectual and spiritual well-being of human beings (Kwiatkowska, T. 2008. *Controversies of Environmental Ethics.* Mexico: UAM- Iztapalapa, Plaza y Valdés, p. 12).

[33] The purpose of the land ethic is to recognise multiple community values and to seek the integration of pluralistic values at multiple levels. This offers a potential basis for protecting and conserving cultural and biological diversity in a socially just and economically efficient manner (Taken from Kwiatkowska, T. 2008. *op. cit.* p. 24.).

the projected growing global demand for food, global agricultural production needs to increase by 60% over the next 40 years (OECD-FAO, 2011). Meat production is expected to continue its rapid growth over the next decade. In the process, the share of global livestock inventories in global meat supply and exports is likely to continue to grow along with *per capita* meat consumption (FAO, 2013), which will represent a major challenge for the environment. Against such scenarios, one promising approach that attempts to safeguard critical natural resources or counteract environmental impacts is certification programmes for livestock animal products produced on farms and ranches that meet environmental standards and follow sustainable and environmentally friendly production techniques to meet growing consumer concerns about the environment, health, animal welfare and other ethical issues (Ibrahim *etal.,* 2010).

Traditionally, humans simply let their herds graze on natural areas; the land was not ploughed and was not fertilised, except for the manure left by the animals themselves. For several decades now, chemical fertilisers have been used, although in more traditional cultures, the use of animal dung is still the best fertiliser for crops, especially from cattle, yaks and sheep. Dung is still valuable as a source of household fuel in traditional societies (Diamond, 1998). It has been estimated that cattle in India excrete about 700 million tonnes of recoverable manure annually. Approximately half of this total is used as fertiliser, while most of the remainder is used as cooking fuel. The annual amount of heat released by this dung - the main fuel with which the Indian housewife cooks - is the thermal equivalent of 27 million tons of paraffin, 35 million tons of coal or 68 million tons of wood (Harris, 1980). If India's sacred cows did not convert agricultural dung into fuel dung, deforestation in India would be much worse than it is today (Cheeke, 1999).

However, in intensive production systems, the major source of livestock contamination is generated by animal excreta with possible presence of antibiotics and hormones, as well as fertilisers and pesticides used on crops for animal feed production. This consequently also affects freshwater replenishment (FAO, 2013), in addition to the mortality problem; it is known that currently around 700,000 people die each year from drug-resistant infections (FAO, 2017).

Regarding the role of livestock in the emission of greenhouse gases (GHG), it is estimated that beef cattle emit 12.14 kg CO_2 e/kg, - for the case of Japan it has been estimated to be the equivalent of 36.4 kg CO $_{CO_2}$ e/kg, - for the case of

Japan it has been estimated the equivalent of 36.4 kg of CO_2 per kg of beef (Ogino *et al.,* 2007), which corresponds to the amount of CO_2 emitted by a car every 250 km (Fanelli, 2007) - sheep and goats, 14.61, pigs 4.45 and chicken 2.84, compared to potatoes with only 0.26 and apples, 0.32 (Audsley *et al.,* 2009).

Livestock make up two-thirds of terrestrial vertebrates by weight, and applied ethology is now helping to develop management methods - such as silvopastoralism *(e.g.* Broom *et al.,* 2013; Galindo *et al.,* 2016) - that reduce GHG production and water and air pollution while increasing resource efficiency and animal welfare (Appleby, 2015). Contrary to popular belief, rotational grazing can stimulate more plantation growth and grow plants that help remove carbon from the atmosphere, so ruminants such as cattle, bison, goats and sheep are the only way to produce food on land that is not suitable for crops (Grandin, 2014). Livestock kept under extensive conditions utilise local resources and renew land productivity (Appleby, 2008).

In addition to the environmental impact of GHGs, livestock consume large amounts of water, both for drinking and for irrigating the pastures on which they feed. It is estimated to use 8% of global water; for example, to produce half a kilo of beef, 9,000 litres of water are required. Other species, such as poultry and pigs, take less water than cattle, with cattle consumption being one of the highest compared to other animals used for human food (Chapagain and Hoekstra, 2004). Bread offers about the same calories as a meat burger using only one-twelfth as much water (Singer and Mason, 2009).

In addition to this, intensive meat production is not sustainable, because in order to produce one kilo of meat, for example pork, an average of 3.1 kg of cereals (plant and animal protein) is required, which would be a questionable expense, as it could be used for human consumption. Another way of saying the same thing is to point out that animals raised in intensive livestock farming are not very efficient biochemical energy converters; to obtain one kilo of animal protein in industrial societies, between 3 and 20 kg of vegetable protein (depending on the species and the intensive farming methods used) are used, which could be consumed directly by humans. For example, in 1990, livestock consumed 70% of grain in the USA, 57% in the European Community and 55% in Brazil, to name but a few (Durning and Brough, 1992). In countries such as China, where they are experiencing rapid economic growth, the increasing level of income translates into a shift towards the top of the food chain: Chinese cattle, which consumed 17% of grain in 1985, rose inconveniently to 23% in 1995 (Goodland, 1997). However, among domesticated mammals, the pig has the greatest ability to transform plants into meat quickly and efficiently. Over its lifetime, a pig can convert 35% of the energy contained in its feed into meat, compared to 13% for sheep and only 6.5% for cattle (Harris, 2010).

The FAO (Gerber *et al.,* 2013), envisages among some techniques to mitigate the negative impact of the livestock sector and lessen the effects that are accelerating climate change, especially in Latin America and the Caribbean, the following: a) improving agricultural productivity by reducing the use of extensive grasslands and increasing intensification, b) reducing methane emissions through diets that reduce digestive fermentation in livestock, c) reducing nitrogen emissions by improving diets and manure management, d) financing projects such as carbon sequestration through the rehabilitation of degraded grasslands.

Anders Nordgren (2012bc) argues that one way to mitigate the deleterious effects of livestock farming on climate change would be through a policy of contraction and convergence, reducing animal production and meat consumption in industrialised countries and allowing developing countries to increase consumption. The idea is not far-fetched, especially if one estimates that *per capita* meat consumption is 122.8 kg for the USA and only 3.3 kg for India (FAO, 2012). For example, the European Union offers farmers in developing countries a Rural Development Programme that is not intended to increase production, but to enhance sustainability by including improvements in animal welfare (Eurogroup for Animal Welfare, 2005; cited by Appleby, 2008). Farmers in Wales, for example, receive payments to improve sustainability and animal welfare; these payments do not distort trade, at most they reduce production as one criterion is to keep livestock density low and should therefore qualify as "Green Box" payments (Eurogroup for Animal Welfare, 2005; cited by Appleby, 2008).

It has been argued that a reduction in the amount of meat consumed in middle- and high-income countries would have numerous benefits: a reduced demand for grain that would reduce GHG emissions and a positive effect on health (Foresight. The Future of Food and Agriculture, 2011). Another way to mitigate the effects of livestock farming on GHG emissions would be through a decrease in weekly meat consumption as reported by Raphaely and Marinova (2014ab), or through the application of a climate tax on meat consumption, suggested by Wirsenius *et al.* (2011) and Nordgren (2012a) for the European Union, which, by the way, would be higher for beef and lamb meat compared to pork and chicken, as ruminants are less efficient in producing protein from forage. Other forms of GHG mitigation are discussed in the review by Alonso-Spilsbury *et al.* (2012a).

Food security and sustainability are priority goals in 21st century global policies, to which applied ethology and animal welfare contribute. Meat and meat products are important in the human diet and the livestock sector is central to the development of food systems; understanding animal behaviour and caring for animal welfare contributes to the three pillars of agricultural sustainability: economic gains, social equity and environmental health (Cozzi *et al.*, 2008; Swanson and Mench, 2016; Appleby, 2017).

Conclusions

Although the end does not justify the means, in order to obtain the nutritional benefits of meat, killing animals is unavoidable. From another perspective opposed to Singer's utilitarianism (1998, 1999), raising and killing food animals is right and justified, if one considers that the benefit of feeding a population with meat outweighs the harm inflicted on the animal and provides health and pleasure to many.

While it is true that animals are often exploited and their basic needs for space, movement and the deployment of their species-specific behavioural repertoire are abused, in the vast majority of cases their basic needs for food, environmental protection, health and protection against predators are met. In doing so, we as veterinary zootechnicians are increasingly fulfilling our mission to serve their interests *(télos),* following the Rawlsian approach to the contract and appealing to the **ethics of care**[35] . We abide by our professional code of ethics and further incorporate science, under principles of animal welfare using them increasingly holistically, assessing welfare under the notion of animal flourishing and thriving. In other words, we take ethical responsibility for animals that have been domesticated for the benefit of humans for food.

A wide variety of welfare assessment tools are available to assess the welfare status of animals for slaughter, whose indicators allow the assessor to determine the welfare status of the animals in a non-invasive, valid, practical and safe manner. These protocols include measurements of the procedures, the environment and of course the animals themselves (health, behaviour and affective states, both positive and negative); they are based on science and therefore free of value judgements. They will have to be put into practice and all actors directly handling animals will have to be trained, starting with all professionals handling animals, as well as farmers and animal handlers and rural owners of artisanal production units, so that through their use they contribute to

---

[35] Ethics of care: Initiated by Carol Gilligan, an eco-feminist, it recognises the inherent right of animals to bodily safety and integrity, based not only on their rationality, but on their emotional lives and relationships with humans, as well as the ethical responsibilities of humans to end their suffering (Gilligan, C. 1982. *In a Different Voice: Psychological Theory and Women's Development.* Cambridge: Harvard Univ. Press). According to Nel Noddings, a philosopher of care, this ethic addresses moral emotions such as compassion, empathy and care in response to suffering, but in a different way from utilitarianism and animal rights. Under this ethic, what is wrong with causing suffering to animals is not that the suffering is increased (utilitarianism) or that rights are violated (animal rights position), but that it demonstrates a lack of care, an inappropriate emotional response in the person (Noddings, N. 1984. *Caring.* Berkeley: University of California Press, p. 149).

improving the welfare of the animals under their responsibility.

Animal welfare is an immediate need to be taken into account in establishing their moral status as sentient beings and in our responsibility as veterinary and zootechnical professionals, and also as human beings. Let us accept that we have moral obligations towards nature and its animals because of their value in themselves and because they are directly useful to us both nutritionally and economically as there are a large number of people in the world who make their living from livestock.

Meat is one of the most expensive foods due to the low biomass conversion efficiency of animals. It is the food with the most nutrients in the human diet and its consumption is based on a whole process of evolution of *Homo sapiens, and* on a production system dominated by the industrialisation of domestic animals in large concentrations, which unfortunately, at present, makes it unsustainable from an ecological point of view due to the environmental cost in terms of deforestation, GHG emissions, water consumption and pollution, which means that alternative systems will have to be implemented in the short term.

My intention with this association of ideas has been to provide ethical and scientific arguments to the meat consumer in the face of the moral conflict that this habit causes in society, although in the end I could, like others, defend this habit simply as a *prima facie* preference[36].

In conclusion, I can only recommend that if the reader is an omnivore, he/she should practice responsible consumption and develop the respect due to the food he/she eats, without waste; that he/she should be aware that a sentient and conscious being was killed to feed, nourish and enjoy its meat, appealing to our right to food autonomy.

---

[36] *Prima facie:* Latin phrase frequently used in judicial proceedings, which means at first sight or in principle, implying the appearance of a right or a situation, but without prejudging the matter (Ossorio, M. 2000. *Diccionario de Ciencias Jurídicas, Políticas y Sociales.* Buenos Aires: Eliasta, 27th ed., p. 795).

Bibliographical references

Aiello, LC & Wheeler, P. 1995. The brain and the digestive system in human and primate evolution. *Curr. Anthropol.* 36 (2): 199-221.

Allen, LH; Backstrand, J; Chavez, A & Pelto, GH. 1992. *People Cannot Live by Tortillas Alone: The Results of the Mexico Nutrition Collaborative Research Support Program.* CT, USA, 290 pp. Available at: http://crsps.net/wp-content/downloads/Nutrition/Inventoried%2010.2/16-1992-8-6.pdf.

Alonso, M. 2012a. Pig welfare audits in intensive production farms. *Memorias de las 4as Jornadas de Fisiopatología y Clínica Veterinaria.* D Mota *et al.* (eds.). Universidad Autónoma Metropolitana, Unidad Xochimilco. 7-9 February, pp. 45-50.

Alonso, M. 2012b. Indicators and protocols for the assessment of welfare in domestic animals. In: JJ Taylor (ed.), *Inclusión de Temas de Bienestar Animal en los Planes de Estudio de la Carrera de Medicina Veterinaria y Zootecnia en México.* Mexico: Universidad de Guadalajara, CUMEX, Cátedra Nacional de Medicina Veterinaria "Aline Schunemann", pp. 39-53.

Alonso-Spilsbury, M; Ramírez-Necoechea, R and Taylor-Preciado, JJ. 2012a. Climate change and its impact on animal food production. *RedVet,* 13 (11): 1-25. URL: http://www.veterinaria.org/revistas/redvet/n111112/111204.pdf

Alonso-Spilsbury, M; Ramírez-Necoechea, R and Taylor-Preciado, JJ. 2012b. Status of animal welfare teaching in the curricula of veterinary medical schools and faculties in Mexico. D Mota-Rojas *et al.* (eds.), *Memorias Primer Congreso Iberoamericano de Bienestar Animal y 6as Jornadas de Estrés Animal.* Universidad del Valle de México, Mexico City, Mexico, 5-6 December, pp. 169-171.

Aluja, AS. 2011. Animal welfare in the teaching of veterinary medicine and zootechnics: why and what for? *Vet. Méx.,* 42 (2): 137-147.

American Dietetic Association. 2009. Position of the American Dietetic Association: Vegetarian diets. *J. Am. Diet Assoc.,* 109: 1266-1282.

Appleby, MC. 2008. Animals and people first. *RedVet,* 9(10B): 1-6.

Appleby, MC. 2015. Applied ethology for ever: animal management and welfare are integral to sustainability. T Yasue. S Ito, S Ninomiya, K Uetake and S Morita (eds.), *Proc. of the 49th[th] Congress of the International Society for Applied Ethology.* The Netherlands: Wageningen Acad. Pub., 14-17 Sept., Sapporo, Japan, p. 40.

Appleby, MC. 2017. Understanding human and other animal behaviour: ethology, welfare and food policy. MB Jensen *et al.* (eds.), *Proc. of the 51th[th] Congress of the International Society for Applied Ethology,* The Netherlands: Wageningen Acad. Pub., 7-10th[th] Aug., Arhus, Denmark, p. 46.

Appleby, MC; Hughes, BO & Mench, J. 2004. *Poultry Behaviour and Welfare.* UK: CAB International Pub., 286 pp.

Audsley, E; Stacey, K; Parsons, DJ & Williams, AG. 2009. Estimation of the greenhouse gas emissions from agricultural pesticide manufacture and use. Cranfield Univ., pp. 37-38. [Cited by Nordgren, 2012a].

AWIN. 2015a. *AWIN Welfare Assessment Protocol for Donkeys.* 68 pp. DOI: 10.13130/AWI N_DONKEYS_2015

AWIN. 2015b. *AWIN Welfare Assessment Protocol for Goats.* 58 pp. DOI: 10.13130/AWI N_GOATS_2015

AWIN. 2015c. *AWIN Welfare Assessment Protocol for Horses.* 80 pp. DOI: 10.13130/AWI N_HORSES_2015

AWIN. 2015d. *AWIN Welfare Assessment Protocol for Sheep.* 56 pp. DOI: 10.13130/AWIN_SHEEP_2015

AWIN. 2015e. *AWIN Welfare Assessment Protocol for Turkeys.* 39 pp. DOI: 10.13130/AWIN_TURKEYS_2015

Ayala, FJ. 2011. *Am I a Monkey?* Barcelona, Spain: Ariel, 108 pp.

Baciadonna, L; Briefer, EF; Favaro, L & Mcelligott, AG. 2016. Perception of emotional valence in goats. C Dwyer, M Haskell & V Sandilands (eds.), *Proc. of the 50th[th] Congress of the International Society for Applied Ethology,* The Netherlands: Wageningen Acad. Pub., 12-15th July, University of Bristol, Edinburgh, UK, p. 178.

Balcombe, J. 2009. Animal pleasure and its moral significance. *Appl. Anim. Behav. Sci.,* 118 (3): 208-216.

Baldner, K. 1990. Realism and respect. *Between the Species,* 6 (1): 1-7.

Bentham, J. 1836. *Deontology or Science of Morals. Posthumous work.* Revised and arranged by MJ Bowring. Valencia, Spain: Librería de Mallen y Sobrinos.

Bergeron, R; Badnell-Waters, A; Lambton, S & Mason, G. 2006. Chapter 2. Stereotypic oral behaviour in captive ungulates: Foraging, diet and gastrointestinal function. In: G Mason & J Rushen (eds.), *Stereotypic Animal Behaviour. Fundamentals and Applications for Welfare,* 2nd ed. USA, CAB International, pp. 19-57.

Blumenschine, RJ and Cavallo, JA. 1992. Scavenging and human evolution. *Inv. and Science,* 195: 70-77.

Boissy, A; Manteuffel, G; Jensen, M; Moe, R; Spruijt, B; Keeling, L; Winckler, C; Forkman, B; Dimitrov, I; Langbein, J; Bakken, M; Veissier, I & Aubert, A. 2007. Assessment of positive emotions in animals to improve their welfare. *Physiol Behav.,* 92: 375-397.

Bourges, RH. 1982. Lipids. *Nutrition Notebooks* (Jan-Feb): 33-39.

Bourges, RH. 1984. Atherosclerosis, cholesterol and diet (2nd part). *Nutrition Notebooks,* 6 (Nov-Dec): 17-32.

Bracke, MBM; Spruijt, BM; Metz, JHM & Schouten. WGP. 2002. Decision support system for overall welfare assessment in pregnant sows: A model structure and weighting procedure. *J. Anim. Sci.,* 80: 1819-1834.

Brambell, FWR. 1965. *Report of the Technical Committee to Enquire into the Welfare of Animals Kept under Intensive Livestock Husbandry Systems.* London: Command 2836, Her Majesty's Stationary Office, 85 pp.

Briefer, EF, Gygax, L & Hillmann, E. 2016. Vocal expression of emotions in pigs. C Dwyer, M Haskell & V Sandilands (eds.), *Proc. of the 50th[th] Congress of the International Society for Applied Ethology,* The Netherlands: Wageningen Acad. Pub., 12-15th July, University of Bristol, Edinburgh, UK, p. 179.

Broberg, B. 2010. Animal husbandry and breeding. In: *Animal Welfare.* Zaragoza, Esp.: Acribia, pp. 31-43.

Broom, DM. 1991. Animal welfare: Concepts and measurement. *J. Anim. Sci.,* 69: 4167-4175.

Broom, DM. 1998. Welfare, stress and the evolution of feelings. *Adv. Anim. Behav.,* 27: 371-403.

Broom, DM. 2004. Animal welfare. In: F Galindo and A Orihuela (eds.), *Etología*

Aplicada. DF, Mexico: IFAW, UNAM-FMVZ, pp. 51-87.

Broom, DM. 2010. Introduction: concepts of animal welfare and protection including obligations and rights. In: *Animal Welfare*. Zaragoza, Spain: Acribia, pp. 1-15.

Broom, DM & Johnson, KG. 1993. *Stress and Animal Welfare.* UK: Chapman & Hall Animal Behaviour Series, 211 pp.

Broom, DM & Fraser, AF. 2007. *Domestic Animal Behaviour and Welfare.* 4th ed. UK: CAB International Pub., 540 pp.

Broom, DM; Galindo, FA & Murgueitio, E. 2013. Sustainable, efficient livestock production with high biodiversity and good welfare for animals. *Proc. Roy. Soc. B.,* 280: doi.org/10.1098/rspb.2013.2025.

Brscic, M, dam Otten, N & Kirchner, MK. 2016. What is the emotional state of dairy calves and young stock? C Dwyer, M Haskell & V Sandilands (eds.), *Proc. of the 50th Congress of the International Society for Applied Ethology,* The Netherlands: Wageningen Acad. Pub., 12-15th July, University of Bristol, Edinburgh, UK, p. 186.

Budiansky, S. 1992. *The Covenant of the Wild: Why Animals Choose Domestication.* NY, USA: William Morrow & Co. 190 pp. [Cited by Tudge, 2000].

Byrd, CJ; Johnson, JS & Lay Jr, DC. 2017. Who's stressed: nonlinear measures of heart rate variability may provide new clues for evaluating the swine stress response. MB Jensen *et al.* (eds.), *Proc. of the 51th Congress of the International Society for Applied Ethology*, The Netherlands: Wageningen Acad. Pub., 7-10th Aug., Arhus, Denmark, p. 132.

Callicott, JB. 1998. In Search of an Environmental Ethic. In: T Kwiatkowska and J Issa (eds.), *The Pathways of Environmental Ethics. An Anthology of Contemporary Texts.* DF, Mexico: CONACyT, UAM, Plaza y Valdés, pp. 123124 and 156.

Camacho, K. 2004. Brazil's deforestation worries scientists. Available at: http://www.brazzil.com/component/content/article/79- july-2004/2005.html.

Castillo Sánchez, MD and León Espinosa de los Montes, MT. 2002. Evolution of food consumption in Spain. *Official Publication of the Andalusian Society of Family and Community Medicine*, 3 (4):

Challem, J. 2007. *The Food-Mood Solution.* NJ, USA: John Wiley & Sons.

Chapagain, AK & Hoekstra, AY. 2004. Water footprints of nations. *Value of Water Research Report Series* No.16, Delft, The Netherlands: UNESCO-IHE.

Cheeke, PR. 1999. *Contemporary Issues in Animal Agriculture.* USA: Interstate Pub. Inc., 2nd ed. 320 pp.

Chigateri, S. 2011. Negotiating the sacred cow, cow slaughter and the regulation of difference in India. In: M Mookherjee (ed.), *Democracy Religious Pluralism and the Liberal Dilemma of Accommodation. Studies in Global Justice*, Springer, pp. 137-138.

Choi, D; Davis, JF; Fitzgerald, ME & Benoit, SC. 2009. High fat, high sugar foods alters brain receptors. *Annual Meeting of the Society for the Study of Ingestive Behavior,* 97 (5):

Coetzee, JM. 2003. *The Lives of Animals.* Mexico: Ed. Grijalbo SA de CV. 108 pp.

Contreras, J. 2007. Food and religion. *Humanitas*, 17: 1-22.

Cordain, LS; Eaton, SB; Miller, JB & Hill, K. 2002. The paradoxical nature of hunter-gatherer diets: Meat-based yet non-atherogenic. *Europ. J. Clin. Nutr.,* 56 (Suppl.

1): S1-S11.

Council of Europe (EC). 2010. Available at: http://www.coe.int/t/e/legal_affairs/legal_cooperation/Biological_safety_use_of_animals/. [Cited by Tjarnstrom, 2010].

Cozzi, G; Brsak, M & Gottardo, F. 2008. Animal welfare as a pillar of a sustainable farm animal production. *Acta Agri. Slov.*, 91: 23-31.

Craig, W. 2010. Vitamin B12 in vegetarian diets. Academic of Nutrition and Dietetics. 2 pp.

Cui, SQ; Holten, A; Anderson, J & Li, YZ. 2016. Tail biting and tail damage in pigs: a comparison between pigs with and without the tail docked. C Dwyer, M Haskell & V Sandilands (eds.), *Proc. of the 50th[th] Congress of the International Society for Applied Ethology*, The Netherlands: Wageningen Acad. Pub., 12-15th July, University of Bristol, Edinburgh, UK, p. 265.

Dai, F; Dalla Costa, E; Canali, E; Murray, L; Scholz, P; Wemelsfelder, F & Minero, M. 2016. Equine welfare assessment: the use of QBA to evaluate positive emotional state. C Dwyer, M Haskell & V Sandilands (eds.), *Proc. of the 50th[th] Congress of the International Society for Applied Ethology*, The Netherlands: Wageningen Acad. Pub., 12-15th July, University of Bristol, Edinburgh, UK, p. 194.

Dalla Costa, E; Minero, M; Lebelt, D; Stucke, D & Leach, MC. 2014. Development of the horse grimace scale (HGS) as a pain assessment tool in horses undergoing routine castration. PlosOne, 9(3): e92281.

Darwin, C. 1984. *The Expression of Emotions in Animals and Man.* Madrid, Spain: Alianza Editorial.

Dawkins, MS. 1985. The scientific basis for assessing suffering in animals. In: P Singer (ed.), *In Defense of Animals,* NY, USA: Basil Blackwell, pp. 27-40.

Dawkins, MS. 1990. From an animal's point of view: motivation, fitness and animal welfare. *Behav. Brain Sci.,* 13 (1): 1-9.

Dawkins, MS. 2008. The science of animal suffering. *Ethol.,* 114 (10): 937-945.

Dawkins, MS & Hardie, S. 1989. Space needs of laying hens. *Brit. Poultry Sci.,* 30: 413-416.

de Lora, P. 2003. Chapter XV. Las otras vidas. In: R Vázquez (Coord.), *Bioética y Derecho. Fundamentos y Problemas Actuales,* Mexico: Fontamara, pp. 283312.

Descovich, K; Wathan, J; Leach, M; Buchanan-Smith, H; Flecknell, P; Farningham, D & Vick, SJ. 2017. What can facial expression reveal about animal welfare? Supporting evidence and potential pitfalls. MB Jensen, MS Herskin & J Malmkvist (eds.), *Proc. of the 51st[th] Congress of the International Society for Applied Ethology,* The Netherlands: Wageningen Acad. Pub., 7-10th Aug., Arhus, Denmark, p. 78.

Désire, L; Boissy, A & Veissier, I. 2002. Emotions in farm animals: a new approach to animal welfare in applied ethology. *Behav. Proc.,* 60 (2): 165-180.

Diamond, C. 1978. Eating meat and eating people. *Philos.,* 53 (206): 465-479.

Diamond, J. 1998. *Guns, Germs and Steel. Human Society and its Destinies.* Madrid, Spain: Debate, 537 pp.

Dol, M. 1997. *Animal Consciousness and Animal Ethics: Perspectives from The Netherlands.* The Netherlands: Uitgesverij van Gorcum, 264 pp.

Domínguez-Rodrigo, M; Bunn, HT; Mabulla, AZP; Baquedano, E; Uribelarrea, D; Pérez-González, A; Gidna, A; Yravedra, J; Diez-Martin, F; Egeland, CP; Barba, R; Arriaza, MC; Organista, E & Ansón, M. 2014. On meat eating and human evolution: A taphonomic analysis of BK4b (Upper Bed II, Olduvai Gorge, Tanzania), and its bearing on hominin megafaunal consumption. *Quater. Intern,* (322-323): 129-152.

Dorado, D. 2010. The moral consideration of nonhuman animals in the last forty years: an annotated bibliography. T¿Xog *Rev. Iberoam. Est. Utilitaristas,* 17 (1): 47-63.

UN. 1948. *Universal Declaration of Human Rights.* Adopted and proclaimed by the General Assembly in its resolution 217 A (III) of 10   December 1948   : https://www.ohchr.org/EN/UDHR/Documents/UDHRTranslations/spn.pdf

Durning, AT and Brough, HB. 1992. Reforming the livestock economy. In: R Lester *et al.* (eds.), *The World Situation 1992,* Barcelona, Spain: Apóstrofe, CIP, p. 120 [Quoted by Riechmann, 2000].

Ehrlich, A. 1964. Neural control of feeding behavior. *Psychol. Bull.,* 61 (2): 100114.

Ekesbo, I. 2010. The Swedish proposal. In: *Animal Welfare.* Zaragoza, Spain: Acribia, pp. 179-191.

EU Directive 2008/120/EC. Official Journal of the European Union.

Eurogroup for Animal Welfare. 2005. Eurogroup for Animal Welfare 2005 into the fold: Creating Incentives for Improved Animal Welfare under the Rural Development Regulation. Eurogroup for Animal Welfare, Brussels, Belgium [Cited by Appleby, 2007].

European Commission (EC). 2007. Treaty of Lisbon amending the Treaty on European Union and the Treaty establishing the European Community, signed at Lisbon, 13 December 2007. [Cited by Tjarnstrom, 2010].

European Union. 1997. Treaty of Amsterdam amending the Treaty on European Union, the Treaties establishing the European Communities and certain related acts. Protocol annexed to the Treaty of the European Community. Protocol on protection and welfare of animals. *Office J. Euro. Communities C 340,* 10/11/1997, 110 pp.

Fanelli, D. 2007. Meat is murder on the environment. *New Scientist,* 195 (2613): 115. [Cited by Nordgren, 2009].

FAO/WHO/UNU. 1991. *Energy and protein requirements.* Report of a Joint Expert Consultation. WHO Technical Report Series 724. Geneva, Switzerland: World Health Organization. Food and Agriculture Organization of the United Nations, United Nations University   : http://www.fao.org/docrep/003/aa040e/aa040e00.htm

FAO. 2004. *FAO Study. Ethical Issues 3. The Ethics of Sustainable Intensification of Agriculture.* Rome, Italy: Food and Agriculture Organization of the United Nations, FAO. 28 pp.

FAO. 2006. *Livestock Livestock's Long Shadow. Environmental Aspects and Alternatives.* Rome, Italy: Food and Agriculture Organization of the United Nations,   FAO.   Available   at: http://www.fao.org/newsroom/es/news/2006/1000448/index.html.

FAO. 2009. *The State of Food and Agriculture. Livestock under Review.* Rome, Italy: Food and Agriculture Organization of the United Nations, FAO. 184 pp. Available at: https://www.fao.org.br/download/i0680s.pdf.

FAO. 2012. Statistics. Food and Agriculture Organization, Rome, Italy. Available at: http://faostat.fao.org/site/610/DesktopDefault.aspx?PageID=610#ancor.

FAO. 2013. *The State of Food and Agriculture. Food Systems for Better Nutrition.* Rome, Italy: Food and Agriculture Organization of the United Nations, FAO, 109 pp.

FAO. 2017. *The Future of Food and Agriculture. Trends and Challenges. Abridged Version*. Rome, Italy: Food and Agriculture Organization of the United Nations, FAO, 47 pp. Available at: www.fao.org/3/a-i6583e.pdf

FAWC. 1993. *Second Report on Priorities for Research and Development in Farm Animal Welfare*. London, UK: Farm Animal Welfare Council, Ministry of Fisheries and Food.

FedMVZ. 1999. *Código de Ética Profesional del Médico Veterinario y Zootecnista en México*. Mexico: Federación de Colegios y Asociaciones de Médicos Veterinarios Zootecnistas de México, AC.

Fessler, DMT & Navarrete, CD. 2003. Meat is good to taboo. *J. Cogn. Culture,* 3 (1): 1-40. [Cited by Herzog, 2012].

Fink, CK. 2011. The predation argument. *Agora,* 30 (2): 135-146.

Flail, GJ. 2011. Why "flexitarian" was a word of the year: Carno-phallogocentrism and the lexicon of the vegetable-based diets. *Int. J. Human. Social Sci.,* 1 (12): 83-92.

Foresight. *The Future of Food and Agriculture*. 2011. Executive summary. Government Office for Science (GOS), London, UK. 40 pp.

Frey, RG. 1983. *Rights, Killing, and Suffering: Moral Vegetarianism and Applied Ethics.* Oxford: Basil Blackwell, 256 pp.

Friel, M; Kunc, HP; Griffin, K; Asher, L & Collins, LM. 2016. Is mood state reflected in the acoustic parameters of pig vocalisations? C Dwyer, M Haskell & V Sandilands (eds.), *Proc. of the 50th[th] Congress of the International Society for Applied Ethology,* The Netherlands: Wageningen Acad. Pub., 12-15th July, University of Bristol, Edinburgh, UK, p. 190.

Fureix, C. 2016. Using anhedonia to measure negative affective states in non-human animals. *Measuring Animal Emotion Workshop,* July 12th , University of Bristol, Edinburgh, UK.

Galindo, MF. 2012. Animal welfare in university curricula. In: JJ Taylor (ed.), *Bienestar Animal. Inclusion of Animal Welfare Issues in the Curricula of Veterinary Medicine and Zootechnics in Mexico*. Mexico: University of Guadalajara, Consortium of Mexican Universities, pp. 187-194.

Galindo, F and Manteca, X. 2016. Scientific evaluation of animal welfare. In: D Mota, SM Huertas, I Guerrero and ME Trujillo (eds.), *Bienestar Animal. A Global Vision in Ibero-America*. Spain: Elsevier, pp. 191-198.

Galindo, F; Améndola, L; Solorio, J; Ku-Vera, J; Améndola-Massioti, R & Zarza, H. 2016. Behavioural indicators of cattle welfare in silvopastoral systems in the tropics of Mexico. C Dwyer, M Haskell & V Sandilands (eds.), *Proc. of the 50th[th] Congress of the International Society for Applied Ethology,* The Netherlands: Wageningen Acad. Pub., 12-15th July, University of Bristol, Edinburgh, UK, p. 438.

Gallo, C. 2015. Implementation of OIE standards for the transport of animals for human consumption. *Memorias III Encuentro Internacional de Investigadores en Bienestar Animal*. 27-28 October, Ciudad Universitaria, Mexico City. OIE Collaborating Centre on Animal Welfare and Livestock Production Systems Mexico-Uruguay-Chile.

Gallo, C and Tadich, N. 2008. Animal welfare and meat quality during pre-slaughter handling in cattle. *RedVet,* 9 (10): 1-18.

Gerber, PJ; Henderson, B and Makkar, HPS. 2013. *Mitigation of Greenhouse Gas Emissions in Livestock Production. A Review of Technical Options for Reducing Non-CO2 Gas Emissions*. Rome, Italy: Food and Agriculture Organization of the

United Nations, FAO, 231 pp. Available at: http://www.fao.org/docrep/019/i3288s/i3288s.pdf.

Gerren, A. 2012. A comparison of the impact of plant-based and meat-based diets on overall general well-being. USA: Palm Beach State College, 18 pp. Availablein : http://www.palmbeachstate.edu/honors/Documents/AndrewGerren_Sabiduri_a-Submission.pdf

Ginzburg, A. 1996. The beginnings of domestication: Osteological criteria for the identification of domesticated mammals in archeological sites. *Israel J. Vet. Med,* 51 (2): 83-92.

Gleerup, KB; Forkman, B; Lindegaard, C & Andersen, PH. 2014. Facial expressions as a tool for pain recognition in horses. *Proc. 10^h International Equitation Science Conf.,* 6-9th Aug, Aarhus University, Denmark, p. 64.

Gold, M. 2004. *The Global Benefits of Eating Less Meat. A Report for Compassion in World Farming Trust.* UK: CWFT, 76 pp. Available at: http://www.ciwf.org.uk/eatlessmeat/ELM report 2004.pdf

Goodall, J. and Bekoff, M. 2009. *The Ten Commandments for Sharing the Planet with the Animals We Love.* Barcelona, Spain: Paidós Contexts, 210 pp.

Goodland, R. 1997. Environmental sustainability in agriculture: diet matters. *Ecol. Econom.* 23: 190.

Grandin, T. 2006. Progress and challenges in animal handling and slaughter in the USA. *Appl. Anim. Behav. Sci.,* 100: 129-139.

Grandin, T. 2007. Handling and welfare of livestock in slaughter plants. In: *Livestock Handling and Transport.* 3rd ed. Wallingford, UK: CABI, pp. 329353.

Grandin, T. 2014. Temple Grandin asks is it ethical to eat meat? The Pig Site, 5 May. Available at: http://www.elsitioporcino.com/articles/2501/temple-grandin-pregunta-nes- atico-comer-carne/

Gregory, NG. 2004. *Physiology and Behaviour of Animal Suffering.* Oxford, UK: Blackwell Pub. 268 pp.

Gregory, NG. 2008. Animal welfare at markets and during transport and slaughter. *Meat Sci.,* 80: 2-11.

Grosso, L; Battini, M; Wemelsfelder, F; Barbien, S; Minero, M; Dalla Costa, E & Mattielo, S. 2014. Qualitative behavioural assessment of intensive and extensive goat farms. *Animal Welfare Indicators 3rd Annual Conf.,* Prague, 13-15th May, p. 36.

Gruzalski, B. 1989. The case against raising and killing animals for food. In: T Regan & P Singer (eds.), *Animal Rights and Human Obligations*, NJ, USA: Prentice Hall, pp. 185-188. [Cited by de Lora, 2003].

Halweil, B & Nierenberg, D. 2008. Chapter five: Meat and seafood: The global diet's most costly ingredients. In: L Starke (ed.), Worldwatch Institute. *State of the World 2008: Innovations for a Sustainable Economy.* NY, USA: WW. Norton & Company Inc., pp. 61-74. [Cited by Herzog, 2012].

Harris, M. 1980. *Cows, Pigs, Wars and Witches: The Enigmas of Culture.* Madrid, Spain: Alianza Editorial, 246 pp.

Harris, M. 2010. *Good to Eat: Enigmas of Food and Culture.* Madrid, Spain: Alianza Editorial, 211 pp.

Held, S. 2016. Play as a measure of positive emotions? *Measuring Animal Emotion Workshop,* July 12th , University of Bristol, Edinburgh, UK.

Hemmer, H. 1990. *Domestication: The Decline of Environmental Appreciation.*

Cambridge, UK: Cambridge Univ. Press, 2nd ed. Translation by Neil Beckhaus. 208 pp.

Hemsworth, L; Powell, C; Rice, M & Hemsworth, P. 2016. A measure of fear of humans in commercial group-housed sows. C Dwyer, M Haskell & V Sandilands (eds.), *Proc. of the 50th Congress of the International Society for Applied Ethology,* The Netherlands: Wageningen Acad. Pub., 12-15th July, University of Bristol, Edinburgh, UK, p. 412.

Herborn, K; Mitchell, M & Asher, L. 2016. Thermal imaging to monitor development and welfare in broilers. C Dwyer, M Haskell & V Sandilands (eds.), *Proc. of the 50th Congress of the International Society for Applied Ethology*, The Netherlands: Wageningen Acad. Pub., 12-15th July, University of Bristol, Edinburgh, UK, p. 373.

Herrmann, W; Schorr, H; Obeid, R & Geisel, J. 2003. Vitamin B-12 status, particularly holotranscobalamin II and metylmalonic acid concentrations, and hyperhomocysteinemia in vegetarians. *Am. Soc. Clin. Nutr.,* 78 (1): 131-136.

Herzog, H. 2012. *We Love Them, We Hate Them and ... We Eat Them. That Very Special Relationship with Animals.* Barcelona, Spain: Kairós. 449 pp.

Hill, M & York, R. 2003. Social structural influences on meat consumption. *Res. Human Ecol,* 10 (1): 1-9.

Horta, O. 2012. Getting serious about the moral consideration of animals: beyond speciesism and environmentalism. In: JC Rodríguez (ed.), *Animales no Humanos entre Animales Humanos*, Madrid, Spain: Plaza y Valdés, pp. 191-226.

Ibrahim, M; Porro, R & Mauricio, RM. 2010. Chapter 5: Brazil and Costa Rica. Deforestation and livestock expansion in the Brazilian legal Amazon and Costa Rica: Drivers, environmental degradation, and policies for sustainable land management. In: P Gerber, HA Mooney, J Dijkman, S Tarawali & C de Haan (eds.), *Livestock in a Changing Landscape: Drivers, Consequences, and Responses.* Vol. 2. Available at: http://www.fao.org/docrep/013/am075e/am075e00.pdf

IPCC. 2007. *Fourth Assessment Report (AR4).* Intergovernmental Panel on Climate Change. Available at: http://ipcc-wg1.ucar.edu/index.html.

Johnsen, PF; Johannesson, T & Sandoe, P. 2001. Assessment of farm animal welfare at herd level: many goals, many methods. *Agric. Scan, Sect. A,* (Suppl. 30): 26-33.

Key, TJ; Fraser, GE; Thorogood, M; Appleby, PN; Beral, V; Reeves, G; Burr, ML; Chang-Claude, J; Frentzel-Beyme, R; Kuzma, JW; Mann, J & McPherson, K. 1999. Mortality in vegetarians and nonvegetarians: detailed findings from a collaborative analysis of 5 prospective studies. *Am. J. Clin. Nutr.,* 70 (Suppl.): 516S-524S.

Kwiatkowska, T. 2008. *Controversies in Environmental Ethics.* DF, Mexico: Universidad Autónoma Metropolitana-Iztapalapa, Plaza y Valdés, 170 pp.

Lagger, JR. 2006. Animal welfare and health on dairy farms. *Vet. Arg.,* 33 (223): 190-202.

Lahrmann, HP; Busch, ME; D'eath, R; Forkman, B & Hansen, CF. 2016. Tail biting: prevalence among docked and undocked pigs from weaning to slaughter. C Dwyer, M Haskell & V Sandilands (eds.), *Proc. of the 50th Congress of the International Society for Applied Ethology,* The Netherlands: Wageningen Acad. Pub., 12-15th July, University of Bristol, Edinburgh, UK, p. 233.

Laszlow, E. 2001. *Macroshift: Navigating the Transformation to a Sustainable World.* San Francisco, USA: Berrett-Koehler. [Cited by Goodall and Bekoff, 2009].

Lawrence, SA & Rushen, J. 1993. *Stereotypic Animal Behaviour: Fundamentals and Applications to Welfare.* UK: CAB International Pub.

Leach, M & Descovich, K. 2016. Use of facial expressions as markers of emotions. *Measuring Animal Emotion Workshop*, July 12th , University of Bristol, Edinburgh, UK.

Leitzmann, C. 2005. Vegetarian diets: What are the advantages. *Diet Diversification & Health Promotion.* Ed. Ibrahim Elmadfa, 57: 147-156.

Leopold, A. 1966. *A Sand County Almanac with Essays on Conservation from Round River.* NY: Ballantine. Trans. by Alicia Herrera. 1998. The Land Ethic. In: T Kwiatkowska and J Issa (eds.), *Los Caminos de la Ética Ambiental. Una Antología de Textos Contemporáneos,* Mexico: CONACyT, UAM, Plaza y Valdés, pp. 61-77.

Lidfors, L & Broekman, J. 2016. How are behaviours indicating positive and negative affective states in lambs affected by step-wise weaning? C Dwyer, M Haskell & V Sandilands (eds.), *Proc. of the 50th[th] Congress of the International Society for Applied Ethology,* The Netherlands: Wageningen Acad. Pub., 12-15th July, University of Bristol, Edinburgh, UK, p. 267.

Liu, RH. 2003. Health benefits of fruit and vegetables are from additive and synergistic combinations of phytochemicals. *Am. J. Clin. Nutr.* 78: 3.

Marchant-Forde, 2016. Heart rate variability and the assessment of emotional state in animals. *Measuring Animal Emotion Workshop,* July 12th , University of Bristol, Edinburgh, UK.

Margules, DL & Olds, J. 1962. Identical feeding and rewarding systems in the lateral hypothalamus of rats. *Science,* 135 (3501): 374-375.

Marmelada, CA. 2007: Did eating meat make us smart? *Cognitive Science: Electronic Journal of Dissemination,* 1 (1): 18-20.

Matheny, G & Chan, KMA. 2005. Human diets and animal welfare: The illogic of the larder. *J. Agric. Environ. Ethics,* 18: 579-594.

McLennan, K; Rebelo, CJ; Corke, MJ; Holmes, M & Constantino-Casas, F. 2014. Facial expression. As pain indicator in sheep. *Animal Welfare Indicators 3rd Annual Conf.,* Prague, 13-15th May, p. 25.

McMillan, F. 2005. *Mental Health and Well-Being in Animals.* UK: Blackwell Pub. 320 pp.

Mellor, DJ. 2016. Updating animal welfare thinking: Moving beyond the "Five Freedoms" towards "a life worth living". *Animals,* 6(21): doi:10.3390/ani6030021

Mellor, DJ & Stafford, KJ. 2004. Animal welfare implications of neonatal mortality and morbidity in farm animals. *Vet. J.,* 168 (2): 118-133.

Mellor, DJ & Beausoleil, NJ. 2015. Extending the 'Five Domains' model for animal welfare assessment to incorporate positive welfare states. *Anim Welf,* 24: 241-253.

Michalak, J; Zhang, XC & Jacobi, F. 2012. Vegetarian diet and mental disorders: results from a representative community survey. *Int. J. Behav. Nutr. Phys. Act,* 9: 67.

Molony, V & Kent, JE. 1997. Assessment of acute pain in farm animals using behavioral and physiological measurements. *J. Anim. Sci.,* 75: 266-272.

Morgan, KN & Tromborg, CT. 2007. Sources of stress in captivity. *Appl. Anim. Behav. Sci.,* 102: 262-302.

Morméde, P; Andanson, S; Aupérin, B; Beerda, B; Guémené, D; Malmkvist, J; Manteca, X; Manteuffel, G; Prunet, P; van Reenen, CG; Richard, S & Veissier, I. 2007. Review: Exploration of the hypothalamic-pituitary-adrenal function as a tool to evaluate animal welfare. *Physiol. Behav.,* 92: 317-339.

Moss, R. 1992. *Livestock Health and Welfare.* UK: Longman Sci. & Tech. 420 pp.

Mosterín, J. 1998. *¡Vivan los Animales!* Madrid, Spain: Debate, 392 pp.

Mosterín, J. 2007. La ética frente a los animales. In: J González V (ed.), *Dilemas de Bioética.* DF, Mexico: Fondo de Cultura Económica, Comisión Nacional de los Derechos Humanos, UNAM, pp. 267-288.

Mota-Rojas, D; Schunemann, A; Orozco-Gregorio, H; Ramírez-Necoechea, R; Flores-Peinado, S; Alonso-Spilsbury, M and Guerrero-Legorreta, I. 2012. Chapter 9: Pig welfare during transfer to the slaughterhouse: physiometabolic assessment. In: D Mota, SM Huertas, I Guerrero and ME Trujillo (eds.), *Bienestar Animal, Productividad y Calidad de la Carne,* 2nd ed. Mexico: Elsevier, pp. 155-174.

Mota-Rojas, D; Orihuela, A; Strappini-Arteggiano, A; Caijao-Pachón, MN; Agüera-Buendía, E; Mora-Medina, P; Ghezzi, M & Alonso-Spilsbury, M. 2018. Teaching animal welfare in veterinary schools in Latin America. *Inter. J. Vet. Sci. Med.,* 6: 131-140.

Mounier, L; de Boyer, A & Vessier, I. 2010. Assessment of animal welfare using the Welfare Quality® method. *Point Vet.,* 41 (407): 53-60.

Moyano F, C. 2018. Feeding freely or equally? Solidarity and identity. *Rev. Bio. y Der.,* 42: 89-104.

Narveson, J. 1983. Animal rights revisited. In: H Miller & WH Williams (eds.), *Ethics and Animals.* Clifton, NJ, USA: Humana Press, pp. 45-60.

NOM-009-Z00-1994. Mexican Official Standard *NOM-009-Z00-1994,* Meat sanitary process. Published in the Official Journal of the Federation on 26 November 1994. Available at: http://www.porcimex.org/NORMAS/NOM-009-ZOO-1994.pdf

Nordgren, A. 2009. Animal agriculture and climate change: ethical perspectives. In: K Millar, PH West & B Nerlich (eds.), *Ethical Futures: Bioscience and Food Horizons.* The Netherlands: Wageningen Academic Pub, pp. 86-91.

Nordgren, A. 2012a. A climate tax on meat? In: T Potthast and S Meisch (eds.), *Climate Change and Sustainable Development. Ethical Perspectives on Land Use and Food Production.* The Netherlands: Wageningen Academic Pub., pp. 109-114.

Nordgren, A. 2012b. Ethical issues in mitigation of climate change: the option of reduced meat production and consumption. *J. Agri. Environ. Ethics,* 25 (4): 563-584.

Nordgren, A. 2012c. Meat and global warming: Impact models, mitigation approaches and ethical aspects. *Environ. Values,* 21 (4): 437-457.

Notimex. 2014. Population growth drives demand for food. *La Jornada* Newspaper, Political Section, 11 July 2014.

Nussbaum, M. 2007. *Frontiers of Justice,* Barcelona, Spain: Paidós.

OECD, FAO. 2011. *Agricultural Outlook 2011-2020.* Available at: http://www.agri-outlook.org/document/15/0,3746,en 36774715 36775671 48172367 1 1 11,00.html.

Ogino, A; Orito, H; Shimada, K & Hirooka, H. 2007. Evaluating environmental impacts of the Japanese beef and cow-calf system by the life cycle assessment method. *Anim. Sci. J.,* 78 (4): 424-432. [Cited by Nordgren, 2009].

OIE. 2006. *Terrestrial Animal Health Code*. Paris, France: World Organisation for Animal Health, 15th ed., 698 pp.

OIE. 2008. *Animal Welfare*. Paris, France: World Organisation for Animal Health. Bulletin 2. 69 pp.

World Health Organisation. 1948. *Constitution of the World Health Organization* [Document online]. Available at: http://www.who. int/gb/bd/PDF/bd46/s-bd46_p2.pdf

Orlov, D; Rubtsova, E; Kochneva, M; Zhuchaev K & Bogdanova, A. 2016. Assessment of the fear of human in pigs of the Kemerovo breed. C Dwyer, M Haskell & V Sandilands (eds.), *Proc. of the 50th[th] Congress of the International Society for Applied Ethology,* The Netherlands: Wageningen Acad. Pub., 12-15th July, University of Bristol, Edinburgh, UK, p. 424.

Palme, R. 2012. Monitoring stress hormones metabolites as a useful, non-invasive tool for welfare assessment in farm animals. *Anim. Welf.,* 21: 331-337.

Perry, GC. 2004. *Welfare of the Laying Hen*. UK: CAB International Pub. 446 pp.

Plutarch. 2008. *On Eating Meat. Animals Use Reason*. Barcelona, Spain: El Barquero, 86 pp.

Ponce, E. 2010a. Chapter 7. Aroma. In: YH Hui, I Guerrero and MR Rosmini (eds.), *Ciencia y Tecnología de Carnes,* DF, Mexico: Limusa, pp. 199-227.

Ponce, E. 2010b. Chapter 4. *Pre-* and *postmortem* biochemical changes. In: YH Hui, I Guerrero and MR Rosmini (eds.), *Ciencia y Tecnología de Carnes*. DF, Mexico: Limusa, p. 111.

Prandl, O. 1994. Slaughter of animals with the exception of poultry. In: O Prandl, A Fischer, A Schmidhofer and HJ Sinell (eds.), *Tecnología e Higiene de la Carne*. Zaragoza, Spain: Acribia.

Raphaely, T & Marinova, D. 2014a. Flexitarianism: a more moral dietary option. *Int. J. Sustain. Soc.,* 6 (1-2): 189-211.

Raphaely, T & Marinova, D. 2014b. Flexitarianism: Decarbonising through flexible vegetarianism. *Renowable Energy,* 67: 90-96.

Rawls, J. 2011. *Theory of Justice*. Mexico: Fondo de Cultura Económica, 456 pp.

Rebelo, C; McLennan, K; Holmes, M; Corke, M & Constantino-Casas, F. 2014a. Indicators of pain in sheep suffering from pregnancy toxaemia. *Animal Welfare Indicators 3rd Annual Conf.,* Prague, 13-15th May, p. 27.

Rebelo, C; McLennan, K; Holmes, M; Corke, M & Constantino-Casas, F. 2014b. Thermography as pain-indicator in sheep: footrot as an example. *Animal Welfare Indicators 3rd Annual Conf.,* Prague, 13-15th May, p. 11.

Regan, T. 1983. *The Case for Animal Rights*. Berkeley, USA: University of California Press.

Regan, T. 1999. Putting people in their place. *Theorem,* 18 (2): 17-37.

Reimert, I; Stokvis, L; Ooms, M; Bartels, F & Bolhuis, E. 2016. In your face: indications of emotional facial expressions in pigs. C Dwyer, M Haskell & V Sandilands (eds.), *Proc. of the 50th[th] Congress of the International Society for Applied Ethology,* The Netherlands: Wageningen Acad. Pub., 12-15th July, University of Bristol, Edinburgh, UK, p. 174.

Richmond, SE; Wemelsfelder, F & Dwyer, CM. 2016. Welfare indicators for sheep: relationship between QBA and behavioural measures. C Dwyer, M Haskell & V Sandilands (eds.), *Proc. of the 50th[th] Congress of the International Society for AppliedEthology,* The Netherlands: Wageningen Acad. Pub., 12- 15th July,

University of Bristol, Edinburgh, UK, p. 183.

Riechmann, J. 2000. *A Vulnerable World. Essays on Ecology, Ethics and Technoscience*. Madrid, Spain: Los Libros de la Catarata, 424 pp.

Rollin, BE. 1986. Animal consciousness and scientific change. *New Ideas in Psychol.,* 4: 141-152.

Rollin, BE. 1989. *The Unheeded Cry: Animal Consciousness, Animal Pain and Science*. NY, USA: Oxford University Press.

Rollin, BE. 1992. *Animal Rights and Human Morality*. NY, USA: Prometheus Books, 248 pp.

Rollin, BE. 1993. Animal welfare science and value. *J. Agric. Environ. Ethics*, 6 (Suppl. 2): 8-14.

Rollin, BE. 2006. *Introduction to Veterinary Medical Ethics. Theory and Cases*. Zaragoza, Spain: Acribia, 367 pp.

Rosmini, MR. 2010. Chapter 2. Methods of desensitisation and slaughter. In: YH Hui, I Guerrero and MR Rosmini (eds.), *Ciencia y Tecnología de Carnes,* Mexico: Limusa, pp. 43-85.

Rowlands, M. 1998. *Animal Rights: A Philosophical Defence*. NY, USA: St. Martin's Press, 192 pp.

Rozin, P; Haidt, J & McCauley, CR. 2000. Disgust. In: M Lewis & M Haviland-Jones (eds.), *Handbook of Emotions.* 2nd ed. NY, USA: Guilford Press, p. 642. [Cited by Herzog, 2012].

Rushen, J. 2003. Changing concepts of farm animal welfare: bridging the gap between applied and basic research. *Appl. Anim. Behav. Sci.,* 81: 199-214.

Rushen, J & de Passillé, AM. 2016. Validating play behavior of cattle as a positive welfare indicator: a review of research. C Dwyer, M Haskell & V Sandilands (eds.), *Proc. of the 50thth Congress of the International Society for Applied Ethology,* The Netherlands: Wageningen Acad. Pub., 12-15th July, University of Bristol, Edinburgh, UK, p. 325.

Salt, HS. 1914. *The Humanities of Diet*. Manchester: The Vegetarian Society, 3 pp. Available at: http://www.animal-rights-library.com/texts-c/salt02.pdf.

Sen, A. 1993. Goods and people. Mexico, *Comercio Exterior,* 33 (12): 11151123.

Singer, P. 1979. Killing humans and killing animals. *Inquiry,* 22 (1): 145-156.

Singer, P. 1998. Animals and the value of life. Trans. by Alejandro Herrera. In: T Kwiatkowska and J Issa (eds.), *Los Caminos de la Ética Ambiental. Una Antología de Textos Contemporáneos,* Mexico: CONACyT, UAM, Plaza y Valdés, pp. 199-244.

Singer, P. 1999. On the factory farm. In: *Animal Liberation*. Madrid, Spain: Trotta. 334 pp.

Singer, P. 2009. *Practical Ethics*. Madrid, Spain: Akal, 393 pp.

Singer, P. and Mason, J. 2009. *We Are What We Eat, The Importance of the Food We Choose to Eat*. Barcelona, Spain: Ed. Paidós Ibérica SA.

Smulders, D; Verbeke, G; Morméde, P & Geers, R. 2006. Validation of a behavioral observation tool to assess pig welfare. *Physiol. Behav.,* 89 (3): 438-447

Stafford, KJ & Mellor, DJ. 2010. Painful husbandry procedures in livestock and poultry. In: T Grandin (ed.), *Improving Animal Welfare: A Practical Approach, USA:* CAB International Pub. pp. 88-114.

Stanford, CB. 1995. Chimpanzee hunting behavior and human evolution. *Am. Sci.,* 83(3): 256-261.

Stanford, CB; Wallis, J; Mpongo, E & Goodall, J. 1994. Hunting decisions in wild chimpanzees. *Behav.*, 131: 1-20.

Stanford, C. 1999. *The Hunting Ape: Meat Eating and the Origin of Human Behavior.* Princeton, NJ, USA: Princeton University Press, p. 107. [Cited by Herzog, 2012].

Stephen, L. 1896. *Social Rights and Duties: Addresses to Ethical Societies.* NY, USA: Macmillan & Co.

Stevenson, RL. 2013. *In the South Seas.* Spain: Valdemar, 146 pp.

Stomp, M; Leroux, M; Celier, M; Henry, S; Lemasson, A & Hausberger, M. 2018. An acoustic indicator of positive emotions in horses? M Cockram *et al.* (eds.), *Proc. of the 52nd Congress of the International Society for Applied Ethology,* The Netherlands: Wageningen Acad. Pub., July 30-Aug 3, University of Prince Edward Island, Charlottetown, Prince Edward Island, Cañada, p. 56.

Stucke, D; Hall, S; Ruse, MG & Lebelt, D. 2014. Post castration pain in horses. *Animal Welfare Indicators 3rd Annual Conf.,* Prague, 13-15th May, p. 28.

Swanson, J & Mench, J. 2016. Can animal welfare science have a role in creating a sustainable future for animal agriculture? C Dwyer, M Haskell & V Sandilands (eds.), *Proc. of the 50thth Congress of the International Society for Applied Ethology,* The Netherlands: Wageningen Acad. Pub., 12-15th July, University of Bristol, Edinburgh, UK, p. 427.

Tamioso, PR; Parreira Silva, G; Taconelli, CA; Chandéze, H; Andanson, S; Maiolino Molento, CF & Boissy, A. 2016. Inducing positive emotions: cardiac reactivity in sheep regularly brushed by a human. C Dwyer, M Haskell & V Sandilands (eds.), *Proc. of the 50thth Congress of the International Society for Applied Ethology,* The Netherlands: Wageningen Acad. Pub., 12-15th July, University of Bristol, Edinburgh, UK, p. 328.

Taylor, PW. 2005. *The Ethics of Respect for Nature.* Presentation by Margarita M. Valdés. Trans. by Miguel Ángel Fernández Vargas. Mexico: UNAM, Instituto de Investigaciones Filosóficas, Cuadernos de Crítica 52.

Telkanranta, H; Paul, E & Mendl, M. 2018. Measuring animal emotions with infrared thermography: How to release the potential and avoid the pitfalls. *Recent Advances in Animal Welfare Science VI, UFAW Animal Welfare Conference,* Centre for Life, Newcastle, UK, 28th June, p. 8.

Tinbergen, N. 1963. On aims and methods of ethology. *Z. Tierpsychol.,* 20: 410433.

Tjarnstrom, E. 2010. *Ethical impact on EU animal welfare policies: the example of Article 13.* Swedish University of Agricultural Sciences. Dept. of Animal Environment and Health Ethology and Animal Welfare Programme. Skara, Sweden. Student report 336. 25 pp.

Tudge, C. 2000. *Neanderthals, Bandits and Farmers. How Agriculture Really Emerged.* Barcelona, Spain: Crítica, 90 pp.

Vanda, B. 2007. *Needs and Benefits of a General Animal Welfare Law.* Mexico: IFAW, UNAM, 32 pp.

Vanda, B. 2013. Bioethics and animals. Lecture presented at the *Diplomado de Bioética del Colegio de Bioética,* November. Aud. of the Instituto de Fisiología Celular, UNAM, Mexico, DF.

Velarde, A & Geers, R. 2007. *On Farm Monitoring of Pig Welfare.* The Netherlands: Wageningen Academic Pub. 207 pp.

Vessier, I; Butherworth, A; Bock, B & Roe, E. 2008. European approaches to ensure good animal welfare. *Appl. Anim. Behav. Sci.,* 113: 279-297.

Vestbjerg Larsen, ML; Andersen, HML & Pedersen, LJ. 2016. Both tail docking and straw provision reduce the risk of tail damage outbreaks. C Dwyer, M Haskell & V Sandilands (eds.), *Proc. of the 50th[th] Congress of the International Society for Applied Ethology*, The Netherlands: Wageningen Acad. Pub., 12-15th July, University of Bristol, Edinburgh, UK, p. 217.

Viejo Montesinos, JL. 1996. Man as animal: anthropocentrism in zoology. *Asclepio*, 48 (2): 53-71.

Vinyes, F. 2005. *Meat? No thanks! Reflexiones y Sentimientos sobre una Alimentación Cruenta*. Spain: Océano, 287 pp.

Visac, T. 2013. *Killing Happy Animals: Explorations in Utalitarian Ethics*. NY, USA: The Palgrave Macmillan Animal Ethic Series.

Walker, P; Rhubart-Berg, P; McKenzie, S; Kelling, K & Lawrence, R. 2005. Public health implications of meat production and consumption. *Public Health Nutr.*, 8 (4): 348-356.

Wallgren, T; Westin, R & Gunnarsson, S. 2016. Raising undocked pigs: straw, tail biting and management. C Dwyer, M Haskell & V Sandilands (eds.), *Proc. of the 50th[th] Congress of the International Society for Applied Ethology*, The Netherlands: Wageningen Acad. Pub., 12-15th July, University of Bristol, Edinburgh, UK, p. 268.

Weary, DM; Niel, L; Flower, FC & Fraser, D. 2006. Identifying and preventing pain in animals. *Appl. Anim. Behav. Sci.*, 100: 64-76.

Weeks, C & Butterworth, A. 2004. *Measuring and Auditing Broiler Welfare*. UK: CAB International Pub. 328 pp.

Welfare Quality®. 2009a. *Assessment Protocol for Cattle*. The Netherlands: Netherlands Standardisation Institute.

Welfare Quality®. 2009b. *Assessment Protocol for Pigs*. The Netherlands: Netherlands Standardization Institute. 122 pp.

Welfare Quality®. 2009c. *Assessment Protocol for Poultry*. The Netherlands: Netherlands Standardization Institute.

Wemelsfelder, F & Lawrence, AB. 2001. Qualitative assessment of animal behaviour as an on-farm monitoring tool. *Acta Agric. Scand. Section A: Anim. Sci.*, 51 (Suppl. 30): 21-25.

WHO. 1996. Micronutrient malnutrition: Half of the world's population affected. *World Health Organization*, 78: 1-4.

WHO/NHD. 2000. *Turning the Tide of Malnutrition: Responding to the Challenge of the 21st Century*. Geneva, Switzerland: World Health Organization, Nutrition for Health and Development, 20 pp. Available at: http://apps.who.int/iris/bitstream/10665/66505/1/WHO_NHD00.7.pdf

Wirsenius, S; Hedenus, F & Mohlin, K. 2011. Greenhouse gas taxes on animal food products: rationale, tax scheme and climate mitigation effects. *Climatic Change*, 108: 159-184.

Young, JF; Therkildsen, M; Ekstrand, B; Che, BN; Larsen, MK; Oksbjerg, N & Stagsted, J. 2013. Novel aspects of health promoting compounds in meat. *Meat Sci.*, 95 (4): 904-911.

Zanella, A; Canali, E; Lebelt, D, Andersen, IL; Langford, F & de Paula Vieira, A. 2015. An overview of the animal welfare indicators project. *Memorias III Encuentro Internacional de Investigadores en Bienestar Animal*. 27-28 October, Ciudad Universitaria, Mexico City. OIE Collaborating Centre on Animal Welfare and

Livestock Production Systems Mexico-Uruguay-Chile.

Index

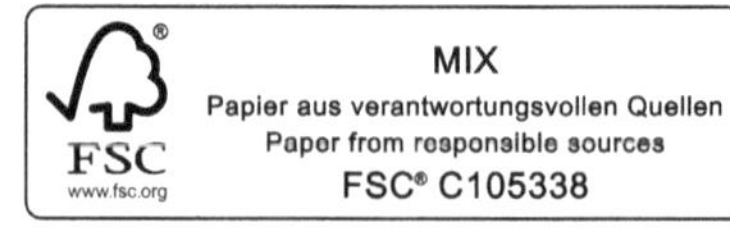

Printed by Books on Demand GmbH, Norderstedt / Germany